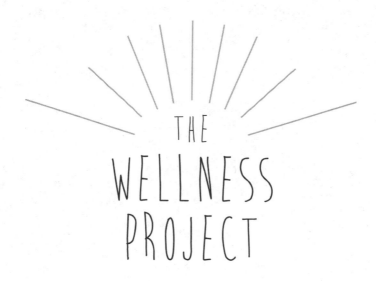

THE
WELLNESS
PROJECT

PAM KRAUSS BOOKS • AVERY

THE
WELLNESS
PROJECT

How I Learned to Do Right by My Body,
Without Giving Up My Life

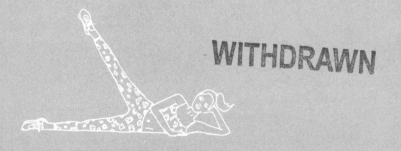

PHOEBE LAPINE

an imprint of Penguin Random House LLC
375 Hudson Street
New York, New York 10014

Most Avery books are available at special quantity discounts for bulk purchase
for sales promotions, premiums, fund-raising, and educational needs. Special
books or book excerpts also can be created to fit specific needs. For
details, write SpecialMarkets@penguinrandomhouse.com.

Library of Congress Cataloging-in-Publication Data
Names: Lapine, Phoebe, author.
Title: The wellness project : how I learned to do right by my body, without
giving up my life / Phoebe Lapine.
Description: New York, New York : Pam Krauss Books/Avery, [2017] | Includes
bibliographical references.
Identifiers: LCCN 2017006705 (print) | LCCN 2017006954 (ebook) | ISBN
9780553459227 (hardback) | ISBN 9780553459234 (ebook)
Subjects: LCSH: Autoimmune diseases—Diet therapy. | Autoimmune
diseases—Diet therapy—Recipes. | Health—Popular works. | BISAC: HEALTH &
FITNESS / Diseases / Immune System. | HEALTH & FITNESS / Healthy Living.
| BIOGRAPHY & AUTOBIOGRAPHY / Personal Memoirs.
Classification: LCC RC600 .L37 2017 (print) | LCC RC600 (ebook) |
DDC 616.97/80654—dc23
LC record available at https://lccn.loc.gov/2017006705
p.   cm.

Printed in the United States of America
1 3 5 7 9 10 8 6 4 2

BOOK DESIGN BY LUCIA BERNARD

For CLM,
my partner in sickness, health, and hedonism

CONTENTS

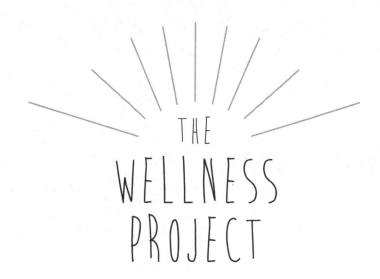

THE
WELLNESS
PROJECT

AUTHOR'S NOTE

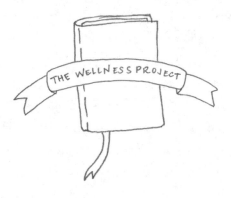

THE WELLNESS PROJECT

Before I Begin

M y illness tale is pretty tame compared to most. There were no epic climaxes in the form of bodily collapses, misdiagnoses, or hospitalizations. My body's unraveling consisted of subtler warning signs that didn't always capture my attention. But eventually they added up to the same narrative through line that all fifty million autoimmune disease sufferers have probably experienced at some point in their lives: why don't I feel *well*?

In January 2015, I launched a yearlong series on my blog, *Feed Me Phoebe*, to help me answer that question. Inspired by Gretchen Rubin's best-selling book *The Happiness Project*, I came up with a dozen short-term experiments that would help me become the architect of my own health, one lifestyle change at a time. And the culmination of that project is the book in your hand.

Anyone who's been chronically ill will tell you that getting well does not always follow a linear timeline. My journey with Hashimoto's thyroiditis started long before I decided to take on my project, but as far as this book is concerned (and to avoid confusing the bejesus out of you), I've condensed the main action into a year of experimentation, while still being true to the ebb and flow of my experience.

Many of the wellness challenges—like my vice detox—lasted a very finite period of a week or month. Others—like rehabilitating my back—unfolded over the course of many months. At times, I discovered that the question I began with wasn't the right one at all. An experiment to eat for my hormones unearthed a bigger issue around birth control; an investigation into the effectiveness of probiotics caused me to grapple with the concept of what it really means to be clean; drinking half my body weight in water revealed how unclean what flows from our tap really is.

While I did treat myself like a guinea pig, I did not do it blindly. I had the help of a very qualified team of professionals. Professionals whose care I was in prior to deciding to write a book, and whose identities—with the exception of my acupuncturist, Heidi Lovie—I felt should be changed to honor a unilateral physician-patient privilege.

You'll find some readily applicable advice at the end of each chapter. These Healthy Hedonist Tips are listed roughly in order of least to most intimidating—basic to niche, point A to point B—to allow you to choose your own wellness adventure.

Which brings me to what I really want to say before we begin: I can't give you a perfect prescription for living a healthier life. You will need to do your own investigations to reveal where your pain points reside, and which benefits more than justify the tough work of changing deeply ingrained habits in order to realize them. Now that I am on the other side of my project, I can say with authority what I'd always suspected: wellness is a journey that starts within. And it's one I feel so much stronger for having taken.

So many people are battling their bodies and looking to others for answers. My story may not offer you a seamless solution. But it's my hope that by following along, you'll be better able to find your own sweet spot between health and hedonism, wherever it may be.

PREFACE

FROM FEEDING ON FADS TO FINDING "BALANCE"

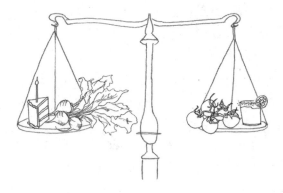

*On being sick, getting better, and paving
a path toward healthy hedonism.*

I'd always thought that bad skin was just an unfortunate side effect of adolescence, that like mouth metal and experimental hair highlights, I would leave it behind with high school. But here I was, a year away from my thirtieth birthday, with a pink pixelated rash around my nose and mouth that refused to go away.

It was mid-December during the winter that spawned the polar vortex and led East Coasters to start sourcing their outerwear from Canada. So I could have simply blamed my face's distress on the subzero winds that came barreling off the Hudson River every time I left my apartment in downtown Manhattan. But this was a rash I knew well.

Perioral dermatitis had been more or less taking up an annual residency on my face since I graduated from college. Every time it flared up, I'd pop into my dermatologist's office for a few painful steroid injections and some medicated cream. Usually, this frontline attack would force my skin to surrender to its former (manageably flawed) state by morning. If it didn't, she'd upgrade to antibiotic warfare.

I had fallen back on these tactics for years without giving them a second thought. But eventually, the shots and the creams and the pills stopped working altogether, which brings me to this particular visit.

"You don't want the medication?" Dr. K asked, her taut eyelids giving me a sharp blink-blink of incredulity.

"Well," I said, trying to appear calm. "We've tried three different kinds now and they only seem to work for a week. Can you please just tell me *why* this keeps happening?"

"It's just one of life's mysteries," she replied, clearly annoyed that my appointment was taking longer than the usual ten minutes she allotted for this type of conversation. "I've had patients with chronic perioral dermatitis for half their lives. Then one day it just vanishes as mysteriously as it came. Clearly something is out of balance and your body is reacting."

This was not exactly the response I wanted to hear from a medical professional charging three hundred dollars for ten minutes of her time. But I knew that Dr. K was right about the underlying imbalance, even if she had zero interest in helping me figure out how to right it.

In truth, I already knew there was something out of whack in my body. My skin was just one outward symptom of a downward health spiral that had been under way for years—I just had never connected the two.

For a lot of us, the first indication that our bodies are not, in fact, invincible, appears in our twenties. And for me, the realization that all those Jägerbombs in college might have taken their toll came when I was diagnosed with an autoimmune disease.

A year postgraduation, after some routine blood work, my childhood doctor told me I had Hashimoto's thyroiditis. I had never heard of it before and was immediately unnerved. The name sounded more like an answer I had missed on my History of the Pacific War midterm than a disease. My doctor casually explained that the autoimmune condition was causing my body to attack my thyroid, a butterfly-shaped gland at the base of the throat that regulates the way our bodies use energy. She told me not to worry: Hashimoto's was fairly common in women my age, affecting as many as fourteen million Americans, and completely treatable with a daily dose of Synthroid, a widely prescribed hormone replacement drug. But I'd probably need to be on it for the rest of my life.

This last piece of news did not sit well with me.

I grew up with a mother who was an early adopter of the organic movement, in a home where "medication" really meant "remedies," in the form of small white homeopathic balls that dissolved under your tongue. I may have taken my morning birth control tablet and the occasional Z-Pak, but being dependent on a daily dose of drugs for the next sixty years was a different story.

That, I would not sign up for.

So I did what any super-mature twenty-two-year-old would do in my situation: I pretended like the conversation never happened and went on living my life.

In the years that followed, I started a food blog, got a cookbook deal, and left a cushy corporate job at the height of the recession to launch a career in food.

I worked long hours in front of my computer, bouncing between tabs of various freelance projects. I hustled hard and took on pretty much any cooking job that involved buttercream and not my naked body. I spent my days teaching nine-year-olds how to bake granola bars and my nights lugging hundreds of mini meatballs to upscale Fashion Week parties where no one wanted to eat them.

And it was all going pretty well, until my stomach—my best friend and most trusted colleague—turned on me.

My wonky digestion was more than just an occupational hazard. I had to stop jogging because I got stabbing cramps after just half a block. I was tired all the time but rarely slept through the night and often woke in a pool of sweat. I ate everything in sight, yet couldn't put on weight, which was nice at first when it meant saying good-bye to the four years of late-night pizza that had gotten lodged in my midsection but became more worrisome when my clothes became so oversized I started looking like an Olsen twin.

It took me longer than it should have to realize that these symptoms—hot and cold flashes, muscle pain, crushing fatigue, weight fluctuations—might be a product of my malfunctioning thyroid. At the time of my diagnosis, I barely knew where my thyroid was located, let alone its many vital functions in determining my overall health. I didn't yet know that thyroid hormones were responsible for regulating body weight and temperature, and that if the gland was underperforming (as mine had been after years of self-attacks courtesy of my immune system), it could affect everything from my menstrual cycle to my sleep to my moods.

I spent the better part of my midtwenties playing catch-up and trying to get on board with the diagnosis I had ignored for so long. I went with a more integrative approach than what my childhood doctor had offered and, in the process, gave up gluten and tailored my day job as a chef and food writer to more health-focused recipes and articles. I read countless wellness newsletters, saw prestigious specialists who didn't take my insurance, and used my professional experience in the kitchen to attempt to heal my body with leafy greens.

And yet, I still felt like I was flailing.

I *was* flailing, in fact. Because despite all the changes to my diet—and all that kale and coconut oil consumed in the process—here I was at twenty-nine with prepubescent acne and a blood panel that looked like I subsisted on Big Macs and Red Bull.

What was I doing wrong?

Sitting on Dr. K's exam table that frigid day, frustrated beyond belief and trying not to cry on her bony little shoulder, it finally (finally!) dawned on me that by retiring her antibiotic Rolodex, I had exhausted my doctor's capacity to find an answer to my skin issues. I knew that I needed to change my approach and that it would have to be my job to figure out what was causing all this external havoc in the first place.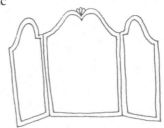

You can't keep running from what's staring back at you in the mirror morning after morning and, for me, vanity proved to be the most powerful motivator.

I had already experienced (and ignored) several wake-up calls regarding my health, but it was the symptoms I saw on the outside that really convinced me to stop what I was doing (which, at the time, I didn't think was all that terrible) and make some bigger changes.

Luckily, this realization came just before the onslaught of New Year's resolution mania. A new wave of health books had just hit the shelves, and you couldn't turn on the TV without some celebrity doctor, fitness instructor, or vaginal steam-spa operator telling you how you could lose ten pounds and live disease-free for the rest of your life just by following their protocol.

The problem, as I soon found out, was that very few of these books offered sustainable solutions. A thirty-day plan for weight loss, yes. But an ongoing strategy for balance? Not so much. Or rather, I should say that they didn't address the type of "balance" I could identify with: the kind that wouldn't require me to drink cucumber juice for lunch and meditate three times a day like the cover girls of the Whole Foods magazine aisle. As far as I was concerned, that type of balance was just another extreme, and I had already discovered that extremes didn't work for me.

The year prior, as I began taking my autoimmune diagnosis seriously, I found myself in the office of a militant naturopath endocrinologist. It only took a cursory look at my blood work for Dr. A to point out that I was a clinically malnourished chef, and the irony was not lost on either of us. Over the course of the session, she convinced me to finally start taking Nature-Throid—a hypothyroid medication made from pig's thyroid. The rest of her solution, however, required a laundry list of dietary labor. No more soy, no more corn. No more cans, no more plastic. No more nonorganic food of any kind. In addition, I needed to detoxify my life, beginning by throwing out the entire contents of my apartment and replacing them with some derivative of baking soda or unbleached cotton.

Dr. A's default approach for new patients was clearly to employ scare tactics, to bully them into making some very necessary changes. Some people who approach habits with more of an all-or-nothing attitude may have had no problem turning their lives upside down overnight. For me, her advice was emotionally and financially jarring. And since she didn't devote the time to fully explain the "why" behind them, most of her lifestyle minutiae went in one ear and out the other.

It was just too much change all at once.

The recommendations I did heed may have changed my cooking for the better, but they also meant I spent more money on green elixirs and supplements than I could afford, and I felt guilty every time I indulged in a Bloody Mary at brunch or inhaled toxic fumes at the nail salon. The more obsessive I got trying to follow the rules that my doctor set for me, and the more failure I endured when I couldn't, the less "well" I felt.

As a chef and spokesperson in the healthy living space, I couldn't help but wonder: if I was this overwhelmed by applying healthy practices to my life, how lost must everyone else be feeling?

I had so many leg ups that should have made my journey easier: I live in New York City with access to top experts and medical professionals. I don't have a family to feed, so I was able to funnel what money I could into my own self-care. I grew up privileged, with an organic-minded mother who fed me bowls of millet instead of Easy Mac. And now it was actually my day job to make those bowls taste less like something that would be served to Oliver Twist.

I knew there had to be a way to ease my body's issues and still indulge in my more hedonistic, boozy brunch–loving behavior. I had to figure out a protocol that would help me discover what it really took to be well. And not just healthy on paper, but to *feel* well—to do right by my body without giving up my life.

If no doctor or diet book had an action plan that actually felt actionable, I would create one for myself.

Having a rotating list of medical professionals over the years in some ways was a crutch that prevented me from doing my own due diligence around my disease. I wanted to better understand my body's specific set of needs—the aspects of my Hashimoto's that hadn't been properly explained in thirty-minute visits with my endocrinologist or one-off listicles on wellness websites. But I also wanted to take a step back and distill the most basic and important variables of anyone's health equation—to discover the nonnegotiables before I got caught up in another round of minutiae.

So instead of poring over studies on how eating more turmeric might prevent cancer, or articles on why biking for twenty minutes every day could lengthen my life span, I began by tracking down experts I'd gotten to know over the years on all sides of the wellness space—yogis, health

coaches, aestheticians, nutritionists, chefs, endocrinologists, gastroenterologists, and so on—and asked them all the same question:

> *If you could tell someone to make just* one *lifestyle change that*
> *would have a profound effect on their general well-being, what*
> *would it be?*

The answers I got to my One Big Question (henceforth referred to as
the OBQ) were surprising. People stopped talking about SoulCycle and
superfoods and started talking about the bigger picture.

With these responses, I started designing a set of short-term challenges to help me tackle each of my problem areas, one by one. The
idea was to dedicate a year to overhauling my health—like Gretchen
Rubin did for her happiness—with
experiments for everything from
cleaning up my makeup to forming
better hydration habits to feeding my
microbiome.

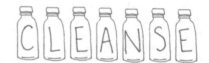

And thus *The Wellness Project* was born.

When I started talking about my project with friends and the readers
of my blog, *Feed Me Phoebe*, it became clear that "wellness" was a rather
polarizing term. While many said that they embraced it, others reported
that they felt the word was elitist and had come to stand for hundred-
dollar-a-day juice cleanses and designer yoga mats instead of integrative
health.

I needed to settle on a definition outside the modern marketing machine, and the one that spoke to me most was from the National Wellness Institute. It states that wellness is "an active process of becoming
aware of and making choices toward a more successful existence."

I liked this idea of an *active process*—that wellness itself was a journey,
not a destination. Because what I'd found that so many health experts,

and even my own physicians, fail to acknowledge is that change is pretty fucking hard.

The struggle is *real*.

Ninety-two percent of people who set New Year's resolutions in 2014 failed to keep them. Why? One reason might be because the objectives were too ambitious. With so many new rules added to the mix every year—usually, the villainizing of one ingredient or another—it's all too easy to throw fifteen balls (or organic apples) in the air and watch them come crashing down.

Working as a culinary instructor had shown me firsthand the failures that can result in the kitchen when you bite off more than you can chew, and tackling these "life recipes" would be no different. I had already struggled to implement the far-reaching advice that my doctor had handed to me without a road map. The grander my intentions, the more I would need a framework for execution.

And without one, the more likely I would be to end up with organic applesauce all over the floor.

The American Psychological Association recommends that you approach lifestyle changes in baby steps, one habit at a time. So for my wellness curriculum, I decided to compartmentalize my endeavors as much as I could. Like the 92 percent of well-meaning Americans, I had already tried to do too much at one time and felt like a failure when overwhelm set in and, instead, I did nothing at all. Isolating each change would help me measure its true impact and see which ones were worth the time, money, and energy going forward.

I ruled out prohibitions that were too crazy or unrealistic. For example, I wasn't going to throw out my entire wardrobe because the clothes contained toxic dyes. Everyone has a limit or an exemption clause, and I put my peep toe–heeled foot down at wearing a shapeless hemp tunic down Fifth Avenue.

To get the most difficult stuff out of the way, while my resolve was at its firmest, I would start by confronting my three biggest vices: sugar, caffeine, and alcohol. Since the state of my skin was one of my chief barometers for success, I would explore greener ways to care for it next. And because our food choices loom the largest, I knew I needed to figure out once and for all what rules should prevail in the kitchen.

Water, sleep, and exercise were basic imperatives that came up again and again in the answers to my OBQ, and they too would get a deeper dive. I blamed my failure on the fitness front on back pain and digestion problems, so I knew that I would have to tackle those two issues as well. And part of putting all the pieces of my wellness puzzle together would be to better understand how to support my hormones. Finally, since physical problems are often driven by emotional ones, I would have to get my stress in check. After all, one of my main motivations for taking on this project was that desperately trying to be "healthy" was causing me anxiety.

As for the new rules and routines I would live by, I gave myself the freedom to modify them as I figured out which experiments improved my life and which, despite the best scientific and spiritual intentions, just didn't. I would certainly measure my progress by internal (blood work) and external (skin) evidence of change. But my intention was not to become the healthiest person on the planet. I wanted to discover a new path forward that I could stay on indefinitely, for the long haul.

And part of that was addressing something I'd always felt was missing from other health protocols: hedonism.

Now when I say "hedonism," I'm not talking about drinking chalices of wine while a servant fans me with palm leaves—though that obviously sounds like a wonderful way to spend a Sunday afternoon. Rather, my definition of hedonism stands for everything that lifts our spirits and brings us pleasure. Restrictive dieting may pull off the pounds and bring us closer to looking like a Greek goddess. It may even make us healthier on paper. But it can often get in the way of living.

I knew that my own pursuit of wellness thus far had been the most soul-crushing when it prevented me from spending quality time with the people I loved. Healthy choices can't happen in a vacuum. And fitting them into your life is even trickier when you share your life with another person.

At the time of that ill-fated visit to my dermatologist Dr. K's office, Charlie and I had been dating for just a few months. My skin decided to revolt shortly after he entered the picture, which only added insult to injury and frayed nerves already being tortured by the throes of early L.O.V.E.

Charlie was everything I wanted in a partner, minus a commitment to exercise and an enthusiasm for green vegetables. And as one tends to do during those blissful first few months, we were living the life of the fat and happy. Was this what my skin was reflecting? And would adopting the practices of a healthful hermit pop the honeymoon balloon?

I had outlined the general idea of my wellness project for Charlie, though I hadn't yet explained the backstory—the autoimmune issues, my faulty thyroid, and certainly not the reemergent acne, which I disguised every morning with a thick layer of Clinique Superpowder. I wasn't sure how his presence in my life would affect the healthy hedonism continuum. Could I still have a social life if I drank less alcohol and insisted on getting eight hours of sleep a night? Was putting toxic sunscreen on my body better or worse than looking like Casper the Friendly Zinc Oxide Ghost? Would a BPA-free linen shower curtain be worth the smell of mildew that inevitably came with it? Which of these practices would be naturally rewarding, and which would make me feel like I was taking an infrared sauna in hell?

These are the daily negotiations we all make, the hedonism points that need to be tallied to figure out if our healthy choices are worth it.

Above all, I hoped that my project would help me find this happy medium—that by peeling away the layers of my body's issues like an onion, I could get to the core of what I needed to do in order to wake up with energy and be excited to take on the world.

In the months that followed my visit to the dermatologist's office, I found myself diving headfirst down the rabbit hole of healthy living. I befriended wellness experts, researched best practices, battled food cravings (and myself), and slowly made over my world, one challenge at a time.

This book is the story of how I did it. And it starts by paying homage to a most undervalued organ.

DRUNK IN LOVE...WITH MY LIVER

THE VICE DETOX

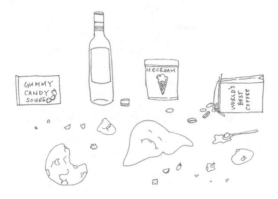

On whether life without alcohol, caffeine, and sugar is a life worth living.

Living with my liver in mind might not have been the first thing on my wellness to-do list if it hadn't been for an organ "aha" moment that happened a few weeks after I left my dermatologist Dr. K's office.

I had just started formulating a plan for my year of experiments when the wellness rabbit hole spat me out at the doorstep of Gloria the Healer.

On a cold Wednesday morning, I arrived at a small walk-up apartment building in Queens. The buzzer for the garden unit had no name next to it, and as I looked for signs of life inside, I worried that my fifty-minute commute might have taken me to the wrong place. Just as I was about to re-consult (and curse) Apple Maps, a mop of brown curly hair appeared behind the frosted glass.

Gloria greeted me briskly as I followed her through the emerald-green carpeted hallway into her apartment.

"Take a seat," she said, motioning to a couch on one side of the living room, which was separated from the rest of the studio by a cream-colored sheet. The space was sparsely decorated, but not in the usual Zen/New Age sort of way. There were no Japanese hanging scrolls or potted bamboo plants. Instead, small wire animal sculptures perched on the few available surfaces. As I removed my shoes, I noticed a faint cat food smell and the prelude to an allergic reaction around my corneas.

After my final failed experience with conventional dermatology, I had reached out to my extended wellness circle to point me toward a naturopath who specialized in skin issues. Some green beauty aficionados offered recommendations for aestheticians who might help calm things down on the surface, but I needed someone who could uncover what was out of balance on the inside—to find the root cause that Dr. K wasn't equipped to investigate. Finally, a friend sent a long glowing email saying that I had to go see her healer, Gloria.

I'd never been one to shy away from nontraditional medicine. Aside from Dr. K, I had migrated most of my health "team" to practices that specialized in more integrative care. But I was still a little wary of the job title "healer"—if it didn't even occupy a listing category on Yelp, it felt a little too woo-woo for me. I was desperate for answers, though. So if someone thought this woman could help me look in the mirror without feeling the weight of the world passing through my pores, she was worth a try.

After a brief chat about my health history, I lay down on the massage table in the center of the room.

"We'll start with some muscle testing," said Gloria the Healer as she reached into the medieval black briefcase beside her.

Muscle strength testing (also known as kinesiology) is based on the belief that specific weaknesses are linked with specific organs and can signal internal problems like reduced blood supply, chemical imbalances, or other distresses. The process was similar to a soft-core arm wrestling competition: I held my arm straight up and tried to lightly match the pressure Gloria was putting on it, which she did while touching various areas of my body, first with her hands, then with small glass vials of potential allergens. If my pressure weakened significantly, she'd push my arm all the way down to the table as an indicator that I had lost that round and whatever she had tried on me had hit a nerve. Or, in my case, a liver fungus.

After the diagnostic was complete, Gloria said she suspected that my liver was in distress due to some sort of critter or overgrowth. She did a few more tests and found a combination of three herbal supplements that seemed to restore my strength when placed on my abdomen. The first was to increase bile to the liver, the second was to detoxify, and the third was to help with evacuation. Without the third, she said, my body 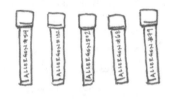 would just reabsorb all the toxins the liver was flushing. "You should also try to give your body a break from alcohol, caffeine, and especially sugar. Those three are like kryptonite for your liver."

I got a glass of water from her kitchen and took my first round of supplements. Though I wondered if the strands of feline hair I found on my sweater might have interfered with my diagnosis, I was relieved to finally have a prescription that didn't need to be filled at the drugstore. Between my friend's seal of approval and the overall body trance I was experiencing from the Reiki portion of our session, I was becoming more convinced that the answer to my skin's problems could be channeled through the hands of this strange little woman in Queens.

No Sugar, Sugar. And No Honey, Honey.

A lot of popular science literature likens the liver's role in our digestive system to that of a sanitation worker. It processes everything—both emotionally and physically—that we put in our body. It does so without bias, treating food the same as supplements, Stoli, and stress. And the work is dirty and thankless.

In addition to sorting through what's coming into the plant, this scrappy organ also manages the storage of sugar and its conversion into energy, produces a vast reservoir of the body's proteins, regulates hormones, and cleans your blood. And when the junk piles up, it doesn't have as much manpower for all these other necessary chores.

If your liver becomes overloaded, excess toxins that aren't successfully flushed by way of the bathroom are eliminated through the only other escape hatch: our pores. And this can cause sensitive skin to react in horror.

After doing more research, it seemed like giving that poor boomerang-shaped Cinderella a much-needed vacation was the perfect way to launch my foray into healthy hedonism. So as much as the prospect terrified me, I decided to go all in on Gloria the Healer's liver advice as my first wellness sprint: for the next month, I would cut out alcohol, caffeine, and sugar.

The following morning, I carefully made my way down the ladder from my bedroom, the four-foot-tall sleeping loft that hovers over my desk. As I stood in the kitchen wondering what to do next, I realized how hard it would be to get my head in the game for the day ahead of me (and Project Health in general) without any caffeine to defog it.

My first order of business was to find a new breakfast ritual.

This is a generous term for what I had been doing in the past. As a freelance food writer who works mostly from home, without an office or even any walls that would help define the ever-aspirational goal of work-life balance, I'd found it hard to adopt any sort of morning routine. It wasn't uncommon for me to descend from my sleeping loft, sit down at my desk while the coffee was brewing, start writing emails, and look up two hours later to realize I was still in my underwear and the coffee was sitting on the counter untouched.

One of my many day jobs was working for private clients in their kitchens, and at eight a.m. I considered myself off duty at the stove. Like most people, I'd reach for the least time-consuming option available, usually a breakfast bar or one of its organic fruit-and-nut contemporaries—anything that began and ended with ripping open some plastic and going to town.

But as I discovered that first morning, the problem with my beloved "healthy" bars was the sugar—or, rather, the honey and non-GMO glucose listed on the back of the package.

The American Heart Association recommends the average woman consume no more than 25 grams (or 6 teaspoons) of added sugar a day. And at 13 grams, one small bar would put me at the halfway mark for my daily quota by nine a.m. With a sweetened latte added to the mix, I had conceivably been blowing my sugar load before the day even really began.

Was it possible that my Madagascar vanilla bean organic yogurt had nearly as much sugar as a can of soda? That the dried cherries I threw on top of it had been sweetened further with apple juice concentrate? And that sugar was even hiding in my whole-grain gluten-free toast?

So much for my breakfast of champions. The meal was a minefield.

The added sugar in fizzy drinks and packaged foods is really the liver's cross to bear because it's the only organ that metabolizes fructose. To deal with the deluge, it engages the pancreas in a complex game of Ping-Pong to control your blood sugar.

When levels are too high, the pancreas steps in and signals to your liver—using the blood's favorite gang sign, insulin—that it needs to store all that excess energy.

"Insulin plays 'good cop' and 'bad cop' in your body," write Brooke Alpert and Patricia Farris, the dietician-dermatology duo behind *The Sugar Detox: Lose Weight, Feel Great, and Look Years Younger.* "It's the good guy when it jumps in to control the sugar riot in your bloodstream. Yet it's also the bad guy because, while it's controlling the sugar situation, it is depositing fat in places you don't want it, like around your belly."

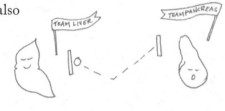

While unflattering for some, these fat deposits aren't always apparent to the naked eye. Being thin on the outside doesn't necessarily indicate how lean your organs are. So even if you're in the vast minority of people who look good in gold lamé spandex, your liver could still resemble Jabba the Hutt.

To make sure my liver would be fully prepared for bikini season by the end of my thirty days, I decided I would try to avoid all added sugar, even natural sweeteners like honey and maple syrup, whose fructose content (though slightly lower than that of table sugar and corn syrup) still gets metabolized the same way as the refined stuff.

One sweet thing I *would* allow myself, though, was whole fruit. When you consume 200 calories of fresh apple slices, the fiber slows down the body's process of absorption. Your blood sugar rises more gradually and, without those spikes, insulin stays out of it. Consuming the same number of calories in the form of organic apple juice, which has the fiber removed, means all that naturally occurring fructose is funneled straight to your liver. Even juicing sweeter vegetables (like beets and carrots) can cause your blood sugar to spike like it would if you were drinking a can of Coca-Cola.

Despite the word "cleanse" being synonymous with the concept of detox these days, I was relieved to learn that redirecting my dollars from booze to expensive bottles of BluePrint beet juice wasn't necessarily the solution to my liver's problems.

Breakfast of Champions

Even with the caffeine-free mental haze, my brain immediately turned to recipes.

Eggs would be the quickest savory option, but I didn't have much fresh produce on hand that first morning to turn a simple scramble into a balanced meal. Plus, I prefer to observe a moratorium on dirtying cutting boards before eight a.m. I considered reheating a bowl of the black bean soup staring me down from the second shelf of my fridge—a recipe I'd been testing a few days prior—but leftovers didn't seem like a sustainable solution for the weeks to follow. As I looked through my cabinets and freezer, I noticed a few bags of frozen berries stashed away and decided that fruit would indeed be my breakfast du jour—in smoothie form.

I shook a generous handful of the rock-hard blueberries into my mini food processor. They were a deep Violet Beauregarde purple but, thanks to the freezer burn that had set in, lacking her plumpness. I forged ahead, dousing the purple pellets with a carton of unsweetened almond milk I'd found in my pantry. Not only would a plant-based milk help me eliminate the hormones my liver would otherwise have to contend with in conventional cow's milk, but in purely practical terms, it was shelf-stable and something I was used to buying in bulk. Drinking your breakfast also offers an opportunity to pack in extra fiber on the fly, like the dollop of almond butter and dash of hemp seeds I threw in as the Cuisinart's metal blade whirred, turning my pruney frozen berries into an icy slush.

Suppressing a few shivers, I sipped the concoction while scrolling through the pile of health and food news that had hit my inbox overnight. I wished I had a banana on hand to add a layer of creaminess, but overall it was satisfying. Ignoring the advice of the white-blond celebrity nutritionist staring back from my computer screen, warning that they were higher on the glycemic index than other fruits, I added a bunch to my shopping list in the name of healthy hedonism.

And then, realizing I was already late for my weekly private chef client, I put the food processor bowl in the sink, threw on my five-pound winter parka, and hoped that the cold winds outside would do a better job than my smoothie of shocking me into wakefulness.

Breaking Free of the Coffee Break

Aside from missing that morning boost, I was most curious about how the absence of coffee would affect my digestion. Had my daily cup made my intestines lazy?

Studies have shown that coffee has pharmacological effects as a laxative, and I'd go out on a limb and say that half of its merry morning drinkers rely on it as much for intestinal as mental stimulation. I had a friend who once admitted that for years she couldn't go to the bathroom without a cup of black coffee with a tablespoon of Benefiber stirred in. (My organs shuddered at the thought.)

The question of what abstaining from coffee would do for my long-term health, though, was a bit murkier. Certainly the research was inconclusive due to many moving pieces that make it hard to prove cause. But individual sensitivity depends in large part on how coffee is metabolized by the liver.

Not only does caffeine cause blood sugar and cortisol spikes, a big downside of coffee is that it competes for precious enzyme resources that are also needed to process estrogen during the detoxification process. This is one reason why women taking hormone replacement drugs (like birth control pills) metabolize caffeine more slowly and can feel its effects longer.

Coffee may speed up the overall commute to Toilet Town, but it also creates a ten-car pileup of estrogen on one of the exit ramps. As a result, those extra hormones get sent back into circulation. And all you need to do is flip open your middle school yearbook to remember what this can do to your skin.

For thyroid sufferers, higher levels of estrogen in the body are especially problematic.

When the thyroid gland is underperforming and becomes inflamed, thanks to repeat attacks from the immune system, it has trouble producing the essential hormones that control our energy levels. This is known as hypothyroidism. Hormone replacement medication is what's most commonly prescribed to treat the condition, and yet many people still experience symptoms of fatigue. Why? Because most synthetic drugs only replace the hormone T4, which then needs to be converted into T3, the active form that gets released directly into the bloodstream to deliver energy to our cells.

The big problem with estrogen dominance is that it obstructs this essential conversion.

The kind of mental and physical delirium I often experienced at the hand of my Hashimoto's made me feel even more attached to caffeine as a method of morning survival. But as I read more about the downstream effects, I realized how my daily cup may have been fanning the flames of my symptoms. It was clear that Gloria the Healer was right to tell me to give caffeine a temporary rest.

To avoid head-pounding withdrawal symptoms that first week, I decided to replace my morning java infusion with a single cup of green tea, a low-caffeine, high-antioxidant option. I knew the headaches would hit hard for a few days and then I'd be in the clear. The big question was what I'd fill my mug with going forward.

Then I remembered something that came up more than once in experts' responses to the OBQ: starting the day with a glass of warm lemon water.

Lemon juice, in general, is one of nature's secret weapons. Its antiseptic nature acts as a solvent for toxins, and though it makes zero sense on paper, when added to water it becomes an alkaline solution. Starting the day with an alkaline drink rather than something acidic, like coffee, helps your liver flush all the junk it collected overnight when it was doing double duty cleaning your blood.

Drinking my first cup felt like the healthy adult equivalent of the warm milk with cinnamon from my childhood—soothing and delicious. It lit a fire in my caffeine-free system and made the wintery smoothie that followed much less jarring.

So a week into my detox, the first hour of my mornings looked like this: I'd wake up at seven a.m., hit the snooze button for thirty minutes, attempt to descend from my sleeping loft without falling, take my thyroid medication, and sip a mug of hot water with the juice of half a fresh lemon mixed in. I would read the news or write emails. Then I'd take my second round of pills (Gloria the Healer's supplements) and make my second morning concoction from a combination of nut butter, frozen banana, berries, and almond milk.

Sometimes, I'd even remember to put on pants.

Making Peace with Prohibition

Alcohol is probably the most well-known toxin our livers battle on a regular basis. But it's not necessarily the worst one, despite what many think. The issue really involves quantity: guzzling a venti macchiato or a liter of soda can overwhelm your liver just as much as flooding your insides with consecutive vodka tonics. Order a sugary, caffeinated rum and Coke, and you've got triple the trouble.

I understood the physical argument for not drinking. I had experienced it many mornings when my body felt like it had been infected with some sort of deathly venom. But unlike my relationship with caffeine, there was a social attachment to alcohol. Even though my friends weren't exactly slapping the Franzia bag anymore, I still felt like some might look at me funny at a bar if I didn't have a drink in hand.

My friend Rob had periodically given up alcohol while training for Iron Man races and eventually found that he felt so much better without it, there was no real reason to resume drinking post-competition. When I asked him what it's like to be social and sober, he found two strategies that were particularly helpful.

First, have a reason.

"For me, it was that I was training," he said. "End of story, everyone gets it. They just think you're crazy in other ways."

Second, if you don't have a reason, have a soda water with lime.

I certainly had a reason. I just hadn't yet learned how to wrap my wellness project into one neat and tidy sentence. The pitch hadn't been practiced in an elevator, let alone a bar, and I was slightly gun-shy. How do you explain the need for a series of health challenges without digressing into the big picture challenges that led to your breaking point?

Hashimoto's thyroiditis wasn't exactly casual Friday happy hour chatter.

With good friends who knew about my autoimmune struggles, I figured I could tell the truth about my year of health. For less-good friends, I could hide behind a lime-studded beverage. And for anyone particularly prone to peer pressure, I could say I was on antibiotics.

"Just make sure to choose the right illness so that people still want to touch, kiss, or share food with you," said Rob.

Good call.

In truth, I was less concerned with people not understanding my motives for sobriety than I was about my own ability to have a good time without the traditional social lubricant. Perhaps it wasn't others perceiving me to be less fun than my own fear that I would actually *be* less fun.

After a long day of work, especially on weekends when I went straight from a catering or teaching gig to meet friends out on the town, I relied on alcohol to pull me out of my exhaustion. Even by myself, with an office that was in the same room as my bed, couch, and kitchen, a glass of wine was often all I had to differentiate work from play. It was the equivalent of taking off my black blazer and sensible flats as I'd done during my time in the corporate world—a symbol that I could be done with the worries of the day.

I wanted to find out what I was really craving when I craved a drink. Was it this contextual reset? The taste of red wine? A feeling of connection? The need to let loose? Latent social anxiety? I set out to identify my triggers, and see in what corners of my life—on top of a bar stool, by the kitchen counter, in the middle of a dance floor—they were lurking.

Drinking Buddies

I didn't even make it to the weekend before I experienced my first bout of angst around the alcohol embargo. It happened the second Charlie showed up at my door.

"The whole building smells amazing," he said, struggling out of his snow boots on the landing. I had tried to compensate for all the new dietary restrictions he would be passively observing by starting things on a very indulgent and positive note: a homemade steakhouse meal.

Charlie entered the kitchen area and slid a bottle of Malbec from its paper sleeve. "I thought this would go well with the rib eye."

My eyes narrowed. When he looked up from searching for the corkscrew, he noticed the laser-like beams of passive aggression shooting from my face.

"Oh shit. I forgot."

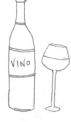

Charlie and I were still very much in the early phase of our courtship. I had met his immediate family members, and we had begun planning a vacation for the end of the year—both very good signs on the commitment front—but in terms of intimacy, we still had a long way to go. He hadn't yet seen my granny panties or noticed my tendency in wintertime to leave crumpled used tissues around the apartment. And I was still acting like it was my MO to put on a black dress and prepare a slab of expensive meat for a casual weeknight dinner. *Just your typical Wednesday!*

Since starting to see Charlie, I had begun drinking more wine during the week and eating more bacon on weekends. We often stayed up past my bedtime and once under the covers, I was kept up even later by the dull sounds of his snoring. I recognized that this was not a lifestyle I could sustain in the long term given my thyroid condition, yet I was reluctant to push back.

As Charlie stowed the bottle so we could share it at a later date, a wave of worry passed over me. I knew that having to pass up a glass of weekday wine wasn't a deal breaker for him. (If it had been, that would probably be a deal breaker for me.) But when it came to my hedonism, I still had an image of the "Cool Girl" in the back of my mind. As Amy, the narrator of *Gone Girl*, tells us, the Cool Girl pretends to love chili dogs and cheap beer, while remaining a perfect size 2. She's hot and understanding and doesn't ever fucking complain.

"Men actually think this girl exists," Amy says, "because so many women are willing to pretend to be this girl."

When I first read this passage, a little piece of my rom-com-loving soul died. It was a rude awakening to my perceived independent spirit to recognize how much my younger self had been swayed by this expectation. You could say that the demise of my two main college relationships was partially due to trying to be the Cool Girl for the precious first few months, until my neurosis and self-respect came bubbling to the surface and I realized it was much easier to just be single and myself.

As I got older, wiser, and more set in my ways, it became impossible to feign a high level of easygoingness, especially when it came to gluten-free fried food and drink. But part of me—that insecure twenty-year-old still lodged somewhere in my subconscious—feared that I had lured Charlie into my love nest under false Cool Girl pretenses.

When we'd met the summer prior through mutual friends, I was already feeling torn between observing my naturopath endocrinologist's lifestyle extremes and having fun. That weekend, though, between all the rosé I drank and the frosting I licked off the flag cake, you wouldn't have been able to tell. Clearly, I had chosen fun.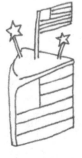

It was the Fourth of July, and I had tagged along with a group of friends for a long weekend at Charlie's family home in Rhode Island. Our host was classically handsome, effortlessly generous, and just aloof enough to make me crave his attention even more than the rosé or flag cake.

As he scrambled to cook a sit-down lobster dinner for ten people, all gathered around a makeshift plywood table in his backyard, he didn't seem the least bit intimidated to have a chef in his midst (even if I was clearly judging his every move). The meal, though charmingly misguided in execution, reminded me a lot of my early days cooking for friends out of my tiny Manhattan apartment. Back then my love of food had nothing to do with nutrients: it was all about the nourishment of the surrounding company and a meal's ability to put your own special brand of love on the plate for all to share. I could see that Charlie understood this. And when he asked me out that fall—to another decadent dinner of shellfish and Chablis—my stomach fluttered with excitement. I had met my match in this food-loving hedonist and consummate host.

Only here I was, six months later, serving him a rich fatty steak with a glass of water.

I had already bemoaned the loss of gluten—the first, and for a while the only, lifestyle change I'd made since my Hashimoto's diagnosis—and what no longer being an omnivore meant for my career. But being with Charlie, going through the early relationship ecstasy of tasting our way through the world together, made me mourn my pre-autoimmune, cast-iron stomach and carefree, college-party ways all over again.

If we hadn't yet taken our relationship to the next level, and I hadn't yet shattered Charlie's Cool Girl ideals (assuming he had them), shining a light on my health challenges surely would. And I might also be forced to consider that in certain areas of my health, and by no fault of his own, he was one of them.

I went to bed with the meat sweats, feeling dually awful.

When Healing Hurts

Two weeks into my new lemon water–drinking, vice-free life, the worst of my withdrawal was behind me. Instead of spending my mornings tapping the keys of my laptop like a one-handed sloth, the other wrapped securely around a mug of green tea, I was now truly waking from my slumber. It was as if the cotton balls had been removed from my ears, the dirty, fogged glasses from my eyes, and I could tune in to the world around me the moment my alarm went off. The throbbing behind my temples that had greeted me at random times throughout the day subsided. And my body no longer seemed to droop as I descended from my sleeping loft.

Since the gradual shift in my caffeine dose was supposed to lessen the severity of my withdrawal symptoms, I wondered if it was mainly the sugar that played a part in the afternoon headaches that pulsed through my frontal lobes, making me simultaneously angry, anxious, and hungry.

I was glad this phase—whatever the cause—was behind me.

Even with my newfound energy, though, there were still few external signs of improvement. I was tracking how the detox was affecting my mood, sleep, and digestion by logging daily notes in my journal, but what I cared about most was my face.

To chronicle the outer progress, I had also been taking a makeup-free selfie every morning. And as I scrolled through the frowny-face pictures on my iPhone, it was clear that my hypercritical eyes were not playing tricks on me. Not only was my skin no clearer, it actually appeared to have gotten worse. A new crop of pus-filled whiteheads had formed along my hairline and my perioral dermatitis seemed determined to become one with the pigment of my mouth.

Intellectually, I knew that things sometimes get worse before they can get better. If Gloria the Healer's pills were supposed to be ushering out my toxins, wouldn't it be natural for some of those bad boys to take an exit ramp via my face?

Only there seemed to be another little problem with Gloria's magic trio of supplements. My stomach had been bothering me for over a week and was now approaching a third-trimester-level bloat. Something would eventually have to give. And of course, that something decided to happen during an afternoon meeting with a client. I tried to smile and talk loudly to cover the gurgling grimaces from down below, signs that my abdominal muscles were losing their battle with gravity.

Thanks to an expensive cab ride and a fierce will, I made it home just in time, and emerged from the bathroom feeling dizzy and weirdly craving sugar. I wasn't sure if this was physically due to a calorie fix or emotionally as a consolation prize for all the gastrointestinal hardship I had just suffered. Either way, I was in no mood to sip lemon water. So I burrowed into my pantry, ferreted out a hidden chocolate bar, and ate the whole thing piece by piece.

Once I had regained my strength and licked the chocolate off my fingers, I called the one person who I thought could help. And it was not Gloria the Healer.

I had met Heidi Lovie a year earlier at the insistence of a friend who swore by her for acupuncture and Eastern nutrition advice. As fate would have it, she began practicing because needles were one of the few things that helped her cope with her own Hashimoto's diagnosis as a teenager.

Though I had switched to a more integrative doctor, Heidi was the first to fully explain that my seemingly unrelated symptoms were all in some way connected to my autoimmune disease. Perhaps it took someone who had lived through it herself to get through to me. And though I only saw her in person every few months, she had since become my most trusted adviser, synthesizing the often-conflicting information I got from other experts and corners of the Internet.

"It sounds like your liver is overwhelmed," Heidi said over the phone as I disposed of the empty chocolate wrapper so Charlie wouldn't see the evidence that I had strayed.

"So this isn't just my detox breakthrough?" I asked hopefully.

"No way," she replied without a beat. "Your liver is totally equipped to detoxify itself without any help. The fact that you're backed up means that whatever is in those supplements is giving it too much to do just to break them down."

I felt a wave of guilt about the negligent way I'd approached Operation Vice Detox. I had been working overtime to become the tiger mother I thought my body needed me to be, but like most helicopter parents, I ended up making my poor liver crack under the pressure of everything I was throwing at it—thirty new ingredients, three times a day.

Heidi advised that I stop Gloria's pills immediately.

"Ugh. My stomach hates me right now. And weirdly all I want to do is mainline sugar."

"Well then, fuck it. Enjoy your chocolate and relax. Your body has been through a lot."

Heidi is one of the few Eastern practitioners I know who is both Zenned out and has a mouth like a truck driver. It's one of the many reasons I like her so much.

On and Off the Wagon

A few days later, I felt better physically, but I was already dreading the emotional test that was coming that evening: my first sober wedding.

I was in a stage of life when weekend social plans became a blur of Rumi readings, tiered fondant, and first dances to Ed Sheeran. And like any celebration, this marathon of love was not a perfect backdrop for healthy choices.

Instead of nursing a seltzer-and-lime, I decided to skip right over the beverage options and orally fixate on food. And this revealed one nice thing about not drinking: more hands with which to eat hors d'oeuvres. My stomach was in better shape, enough so to indulge in the Pinterest-worthy passed canapés. Normally, my enthusiasm would have resulted in at least one condiment spilled down the front of my sole non-black black-tie dress. But this night I had one paw for flagging down cater-waiter trays and one to actually hold a napkin, which made for a remarkably more ladylike appetizer experience.

There were other obstacles, though. Without alcohol (and its subsequent hair tosses and flailing limbs) I was acutely aware of my own lack of rhythm on the dance floor. But the most painful moment of weakness came at dessert. Because of the gluten issue, it's rare that I'm actually able to eat this course at catered events. Most of the time (under the influence of alcohol) I just take to helping myself to a few fingers full of frosting from my seatmate's slice of cake. This wedding, however, had almond flour–based French macarons, double-dipped chocolate-covered strawberries, and caramel-filled truffles dusted in sea salt, all green-light treats for we gluten-free folk.

My mouth started salivating at the sight of them. So I took Acu Heidi's advice out of context and said, "Fuck it." And then proceeded to eat all the things.

Part of me knew that giving in to this temptation wasn't entirely my fault.

We are hardwired to want sugar. It's part of our brain's natural survival instinct to make extremely effective, quick energy light up all our pleasure centers. While other parts of the body (like your intestines) may let you know you've gone overboard after eating a pound of Halloween candy, as far as your brain is concerned, there's no such thing as too much of a good thing.

Our taste buds, on the other hand, are far more adaptable. Though they become increasingly numb to the onslaught of sugar and salt in our everyday meals, they can easily reset once those things are removed. And since taste buds have a two-week life span, I had unknowingly already begun to deprogram my tongue's love of sugar, even if my brain hadn't received the memo yet.

It took only one bite of a raspberry macaron to make my cheeks go concave. The flavor was cloyingly sweet. I proceeded to taste each flavor and, ever the lady, discard the remainder of the cookies on Charlie's cake plate.

I left the party with a throbbing headache, a reverse sugar hangover. But the next day I woke up without the usual post-wedding puffiness, brain fog, and regrets. Even the sugar binge was much more restrained than it might have been under the influence of a bottomless champagne glass. The only morning-after memories to cringe over were my dance moves. And luckily no one else was likely to remember them.

Retoxing

Thirty days into my experiment of forgoing caffeine, sugar, and alcohol, I began to see and feel the full positive effects of my detox. Without Gloria the Healer's supplements stirring the pot and giving my liver even more to battle, my skin finally started to settle down. And it was powerful to see how quickly my course changed once I let my diet alone do the steering.

My overall energy was soaring. For the first time in years, I was starting to wake up before my alarm. I loved not being dependent on caffeine to capture my attention in the morning, even if I was paranoid that my local hipster barista looked at me with a hint of an eye roll when I ordered an herbal tea instead of a ground-to-order espresso.

Getting a good night's rest is essential for your body, but it's especially important for your liver. As Acu Heidi explained, in Chinese medicine, our internal clock gets divvied up into phases that each correspond to a specific organ, and the liver works the night shift from one a.m. to three a.m. This means if your sleep is disrupted, so is the liver's late-night chore of cleaning your blood. This isn't ideal for anyone, but it's particularly problematic for those of us with autoimmune issues. If the liver is not doing its nighttime duties, or not doing them well, you'll have a harder time clearing out the antibodies that are attacking your tissue.

It's not surprising, then, that when my formal experiment came to an end, my nerves kicked in. I didn't want all of my hard work to go out the window—especially when I was finally starting to see results. I looked at Charlie's celebratory bottle of wine and pictured myself waking up twelve hours later, my face covered in a poppy field of hives.

"If you stress about it, that's probably what's going to happen," he said, pouring me a glass of Malbec. It was the same bottle that had sent me into an emotional tailspin the first week of my experiment. Before I had a chance to counter his voice of reason, Charlie clinked my glass and I took a reluctant deep breath. The wine smelled faintly of coffee and cocoa—all my beloved vices rolled into one.

And then I drank.

In the previous weeks of feeling sorry for myself, I had almost forgotten how much I love the *taste* of wine, even more so than the loss of dance-floor inhibition or the end-of-workday calm it offered.

"Has it just been a while, or is this really good?" I asked, one glass in the hole and already feeling my limbs turning to noodles.

Charlie flashed me a sly smirk. "It's really good."

The next morning, I continued throwing caution to the wind with an almond milk latte and gluten-free blueberry muffin. The buttery topping was the first thing to hit my tongue, quickly followed by a river of slightly bitter, earthy brew. The combination made my taste buds do hedonistic hitch kicks and somersaults. It was almost enough to make me overlook the fact that my heartbeat had just been given a David Guetta remix, my hands jittering with the onset of spirit fingers.

There was no denying the pleasure of this combo—nor the deep energetic unraveling later that day that forced me into an early evening coma on the couch.

The Sweet Spot

As anyone who's woken up from an imperfect sleep knows, the first thing you crave after hauling ass out of bed is a quick cup of the antidote. Caffeine is a slippery slope in that way. And it's also one that's very much tied to the other two vices in my detox. Without the morning-after exhaustion from a night of drinking or the post-breakfast blood sugar crash from a fructose-laden bowl of cereal, I found I didn't really need it. Once alcohol and sugar came back into my life, though, I could feel caffeine becoming an important part of the equation again. The key was not getting wrapped up in my vice trio's vicious cycle.

I decided to keep coffee out of the house and to rely on green tea when I really needed a boost, making sure not to drink it after noon if I wanted to sleep well that night. But I knew that maintaining these boundaries was dependent on continuing to limit the sweet stuff.

During the first two weeks of my detox, sugar fully hijacked my head. I was irritable, achy, and constantly thinking about Reese's Peanut Butter Cups.

Many researchers have likened the brain on sugar to it being on hard drugs like cocaine. One French study found that when given the option, 94 percent of cocaine-addicted rats actually preferred sugar water as their drug of choice. But my relentless cravings seemed to be less about chemical addiction and more due to another type of brainwashing: the fact that it's literally everywhere.

Sugar is tucked away on the ingredient labels of 80 percent of the supermarket aisle. It is in every crevice of a fifty-item Thai take-out menu, and on TV, staring me down from the top of a swirling waterfall of Twix caramel. Those Reese's Peanut Butter Cups were perched at the checkout counter of the gas station, the pharmacy, and even the doctor's office. Seeing these cues, I would immediately start salivating, even if I wasn't hungry.

Staying strong in the face of that sugary assault turned out to depend in large part on my new breakfast routine, which seemed to be sticking. For mornings when I knew I would have very little time, I tried to make sure I had something premade in the fridge—a batch of whole-grain overnight oats with chia seeds and mashed banana, or individual frittata bites studded with spinach and sun-dried tomatoes that just needed a quick reheating.

Before I started doing that preemptive breakfast prepping, the thing that conspired most to destroy my smoothie habit (besides the bitter cold of winter) was a dirty food processor bowl. I learned I had to wash it right away, otherwise it would sit in the sink while I zoned out reading the home page of the *Daily Mail* and then rushed out the door. Faced the next morning with that crusty, blueberry-spackled appliance, sugary breakfast bars inevitably made their way back into my life, accompanied by the type of morning-after shame usually reserved for drunken regrets.

During the detox, sugar also crept its way into my meals unconsciously, in the meals I ate at restaurants (or weddings), and, with full awareness, when hunger hit as I was running around the city and the choice was either a quick fix at the bodega or nothing. In one study, researchers found that when people with diabetes skipped breakfast, their lunchtime blood sugar levels were 37 percent higher than on mornings when they'd had something to eat. Perhaps on harried days, when the alternative is a low-blood-sugar hangry meltdown, a little honey or non-GMO glucose along with nuts, seeds, and plenty of other whole food fiber isn't the end of the world.

If I missed sweets less as a reward for good behavior (or unnecessary tummy trauma), and more for the shared experiences, the same was doubly true of alcohol.

Sober dancing at a wedding turned out to be easier than being at a round table as some of my favorite people enjoyed good wine, becoming progressively more "fun" (and telling progressively dumber jokes), while I sat there drinking water and feeling a wave of loser fatigue pass over me. By the end of the night, I ended up craving quiet time with Charlie even more than a glass of wine. I needed the antidote to my self-imposed feelings of alienation. But it was hard for him to hide his disappointment when I made him head home early with me instead of continuing out with the group, which just made me feel worse.

The next day, though, I realized that this line of thinking was just as foolish and unnecessary as a bout of drunken jealous rage. Maybe it was a by-product of spending so much time creating experiences for others around food that I had forgotten about the real reason I had started cooking in the first place. The vice detox was a good reminder that the best nourishment is the company you keep. And the occasional salted caramel ice cream sundae shared with the table, or round of mai tais at an ironic downtown tiki bar, is just the cherry on top.

Social wellness was important, but so was the way I framed it. At the end of the day, I knew that it mattered less whether I gathered around cake or kale, and more about the attitude I brought to the table.

Perhaps I wasn't losing more by not having alcohol in my life than I was gaining. But as much as I was enjoying the hangover-free mornings and the fact that I was now the cheapest date ever (more money for frozen organic blueberries!), this hedonist wanted to find moderation back on the sauce.

One immediate impact of my retox was that I instantly became a wine snob. This was not something I would ordinarily want to be, but it wasn't such a bad thing to embrace in the name of my health. In the weeks that followed, I made an effort to start drinking more for taste—to sip slower, and if that first mouthful caused my lips to pucker, I'd casually put down the plastic cup of five-buck chuck and proceed to socialize hands-free.

I also noticed the times when I didn't miss alcohol, like more intimate weekday catch-up dinners where I wouldn't have wanted to spend fifteen dollars on a fancy glass of wine when there were so many other delicious things to drink up for free. In New York City, it's amazing how a cocktail at dinner can start to feel mandatory, even over a home-cooked meal on a Monday. It made me wonder: How many people out there are drinking just because it's the default? Because it's what Cool Girls do? Because it's easier than fielding judgmental stares or pregnancy questions? At twenty-nine, I thought I would have outgrown peer pressure. But maybe we never really do.

This first leg of my journey was also a good reality check about the true meaning of detox. Healing your liver doesn't require you to supplement with pills, juice cleanses, or anything that promises to flush you in one end or out the other. I had a rough start with Gloria the Healer. But I was grateful to her for holding up a mirror to my own dangerous desperation. For reminding me of one of my golden rules for this project: there are no quick fixes.

It recalibrated my bullshit meter at just the right time and reminded me that diet is the most powerful way to fix inner and outer chaos—more so than any pill, natural or otherwise. I had already felt pulled in some extreme directions in this department by my militant endocrinologist. But in giving me so many things to eliminate or worry about, I ended up toeing the line. The vice detox was the strictest I had been with my food choices in a long time, but in focusing on just a few ingredients, for a short period, I felt less lost and obsessive. The changes were sweeping, but they were focused and manageable. And I didn't have to wonder which really moved the needle.

I felt good about staying off coffee and I would continue to avoid processed foods as much as possible, without staying fully on the sugar-free train. I wanted to keep starting my day with a cup of lemon water and a high-fiber breakfast, be it a super-seedy smoothie or a plate of leftovers with an egg on top. And I knew that even if I found myself with a bar in hand, it was better for my blood sugar than eating no breakfast at all. The important thing was continuing to read food labels so I knew exactly where I stood. Less mindless sugar and alcohol meant more room for the occasional treat.

Even with many fewer weeknight glasses of wine and my own ongoing snobbery to set limitations, though, I knew I had to find more ways to reduce the toxins bombarding my liver every day. The next step was to take my focus from the liquor cabinet to the bathroom cabinet.

Healthy Hedonist Detox Tips

The vice detox can be a huge jump start for your liver. But if you aren't going to give them up for good, here are some ways to find moderation and mindfulness off the wagon.

1. *Don't consume alcohol, caffeine, or sugar on an empty stomach.* A small bite of fiber-rich food (even a handful of peanuts off the bar!) can slow absorption and limit the negative effects these vices have on your blood sugar and hormone levels.

2. *Skip all sweet beverages.* This means soda as well as fruit juice. Even green juices are usually packed with naturally sweet ingredients— apples, pears, carrots—to make the greens more palatable. If you can't quit fruit-blend green drinks, think of them as a supplement, not a meal, and sip them with your lunch for extra nutrients. Better yet, stick with an "all greens" variety that doesn't include fruit.

3. *If you do drink caffeinated beverages, do so before noon.* Caffeine takes twenty-four hours to work its way fully out of your system, which means anything you drink after midday will still be strong enough in your bloodstream to cause problems at bedtime. Swapping coffee for green tea is a great baby step if you don't want to cut caffeine completely out of your life or don't want to experience withdrawal on the road to doing so.

4. *Alternate your alcoholic drinks with water.* Even if you're drinking in moderation, alcohol causes dehydration. Having a glass of water after every drink can help lessen the blow to your liver and slow down your total consumption by giving you something else to sip on between martinis.

5. *Avoid the savory sugar sources too.* Southern and Asian cuisines are addictively sweet by nature. Just look at the ingredients list of a store-bought teriyaki or BBQ sauce and you'll find that sugar is the second line item (and potentially third, fourth, and fifth). Stick with Mexican, Middle Eastern, Greek, or Indian food if you're searching for a sugar-free ethnic meal out.

6. *Make raw honey your (occasional) sweetener of choice.* This natural sweetener was used in ancient remedies for its anti-inflammatory and antifungal qualities. Just remember not to heat it if you want to retain them. I use it for a little extra sweetness in overnight oats or on Greek yogurt.

7. *Take an activated charcoal capsule.* There are times in our lives—a best friend's bachelorette party, dinner with a client, your own birthday—when social norms may encourage you to drink more than you'd like. If you know you will overindulge, take an activated charcoal capsule before you go out. It absorbs toxins and will help your liver deal with all that tequila. It will also mitigate the intoxicating effects of the alcohol, so if you're after the social lubrication, you're better off just limiting your consumption. Charcoal also absorbs medications, rendering them ineffective. So take it at least two hours before or after other pills.

8. *Don't skip breakfast!* Missing a meal messes with your blood sugar and gets your cortisol levels pumping. Breakfast is essential for your daily metabolism. If you don't have time to make something at home, a bar with plenty of fiber and not too much added sugar is better than nothing at all, but Violet's Big Blueberry-Almond Smoothie (page 46) takes five minutes. Hashi Posse: make sure to wait twenty minutes after taking your thyroid medication before eating.

VIOLET'S BIG BLUEBERRY-ALMOND SMOOTHIE

Makes 1 drink

In my quest to find the perfect morning smoothie that's easy to throw together, deliciously creamy, naturally sweet, and protein-packed, I've tried more ingredient combos than I can remember. But my all-time favorite is this five-ingredient blue bombshell. Though higher on the glycemic index than blueberries, a little banana can go a long way to give your smoothie some richness. The natural sugars are offset by fiber-rich almond butter. To put the brakes on your blood sugar even further, check out some other easy fiber additions below.

1 cup almond milk

½ cup frozen blueberries

1 medium frozen banana

1 tablespoon almond butter

Pinch of sea salt

Combine all of the ingredients in a blender and puree until smooth. Add more almond milk if necessary to create your ideal consistency. Pour into a tall glass and enjoy.

HEALTHY HEDONIST TIPS

All it takes is a few minutes post–shopping trip to prep your smoothie haul for the week. Immediately peel your bananas, cut in half widthwise, and toss in a freezer bag. You can even portion out all of the ingredients into single-serving bags or mason jars, eliminating the need for daily prep. Make sure to buy unsweetened and unsalted almond butter so you can control your own sodium and sugar levels.

MARKET SWAPS

Substitute raspberries or strawberries for the blueberries, or if you prefer a green color palette, swap a handful of spinach for the berries altogether. For even less sugar, substitute half an avocado for the banana. If using fresh produce, you can add an ice cube to get your smoothie frosty. For even more protein and fiber, try tossing in 1 teaspoon of hemp or chia seeds. Adding ¼ cup of plain lactose-free kefir or 2 tablespoons of plain full-fat Greek yogurt will up your probiotic intake as well.

GREEN TEA ARNOLD PALMERS

Makes 4 drinks

This drink is a combination of the two beverages I relied on while weaning myself off coffee: green tea and fresh lemon water. Lemon juice helps enhance mineral absorption, which is great news for all those green tea antioxidants. The honey is optional—especially if you're staying away from sugar—but a few teaspoons of raw honey are much better for your blood sugar than the simple syrup in an iced vanilla latte.

....

2 green tea bags (or 2 tablespoons loose leaf)

$^1/_3$ cup freshly squeezed lemon juice

2 tablespoons raw honey, optional

$^1/_4$ cup fresh mint leaves, loosely packed

1. Bring 1 quart of water to a boil in a teakettle. Place the green tea bags (or infuser filled with loose leaf tea) in a large pitcher. Pour the hot water over the tea and let steep for 10 minutes, or until a light caramel color. Remove the tea bags or infuser.

2. Allow to cool for 10 minutes, or until it's cool enough to sip. Stir in the lemon juice and honey, if using. Transfer to the fridge to chill completely. Serve over ice and garnish with mint leaves.

HEALTHY HEDONIST TIPS

Raw, unpasteurized honey contains many nutrients and is considered an anti-inflammatory food when consumed in moderation. If using raw honey in this recipe, don't skip letting the tea cool before adding it.

MARKET SWAPS

Replace the lemon with lime or blood orange juice, and get creative with your tea. I love using a few whole dried hibiscus flowers for a pink herbal version that's completely caffeine-free.

GREEN BEAUTY

FEEDING MY SKIN FROM THE OUTSIDE IN

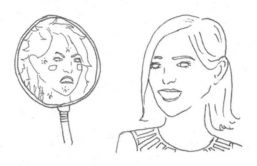

*On starting Makeup-Free Mondays and
purifying my personal care products.*

Before I started my wellness project, I treated my skin like a separate entity.

I tended to forget that my face, whether dewy and soft or dry and craterlike, was as much a reflection of my general health as any other part of the body. My years of breakouts and rashes were clear signs of some sort of internal imbalance. But instead of addressing the root causes—as I finally tried to do during my vice detox—I just slathered on expensive creams to fix my imperfections and heavy powder to cover them up.

I had Gloria the Healer to thank, in part, for finally getting me to link what I was putting *in* my body with what was happening on my skin. Now that my face seemed to be in remission from its flare-up, I was certainly going to keep an eye on how my partial return to sugar, alcohol, and caffeine provoked changes in my appearance. But I also wanted to continue doing everything I could to heal my skin from the outside in.

The irony of makeup is that the less you need it, the easier it is to go without. And the face that we feel most embarrassed to show the world has the skin that could probably benefit from not being covered up all the time.

Though I knew a breather from irritating sponges and spackle could only help matters, I wasn't sure I was ready yet to completely put down my powder. As a baby step, I decided the next thing on my wellness agenda would be to cut the cord with my makeup for just one day a week.

Every substance we put on our skin gets absorbed into our bodies, sometimes within seconds (just think of a nicotine patch). According to a survey by the Environmental Working Group, women use an average of twelve personal-care products, imposing around 168 unique ingredients on our livers on a daily basis. The idea of consuming that many different chemicals in one meal seems crazy. So why is it more acceptable to ambush our insides via our skin?

The more research I did on my Hashimoto's, the more I realized that everything I'd been doing to conceal my outer chaos was potentially contributing to its internal causes. Going through laundry lists of the most offending additives and their side effects was enough to make anyone want to head to the kitchen and start making soap out of shea butter and goat milk. More than one in five personal-care products contain chemicals suspected of causing cancer. And 60 percent of conventional makeup products include known endocrine disruptors on their ingredients lists. These substances mimic sex hormones in the body and can cause a host of reproductive issues, hormone imbalances, and other conditions—not to mention exacerbate those (like my Hashimoto's) that already exist.

As the wise twenty-first-century philosopher Beyoncé once said: Pretty hurts.

For the sake of my struggling liver and defective thyroid, I wanted to take the leap and switch my products to more natural options—even if I might have gotten more liquid courage from my concealer than from a glass of wine.

Makeup-Free Mondays

I first heard of Makeup-Free Mondays through my friend Alexis Wolfer, who launched the campaign on her website, The Beauty Bean, as a way for women to embrace their natural beauty and be more comfortable in their skin. She's even gotten celebrities like Brooklyn Decker and Giada De Laurentiis to join the movement by sharing their bare-faced selfies with the world.

A growing list of dermatologists also recommend taking a break from makeup in an effort to promote healthier, more youthful-looking skin. Parabens and other chemicals in conventional products accumulate in the skin's outermost layers, leading to the breakdown of collagen and elastin, which are essential for keeping skin firm, supple, and springy. Giving your face a breather from these ingredients allows those skin cells to turn over and regenerate, something no amount of makeup remover can do.

I loved the idea of allowing my face time to heal one day a week, but I knew that the experiment wouldn't necessarily be an easy one emotionally.

When my skin was at its worst, I went to great lengths to ensure that Charlie didn't see my crater-faced truth. On the nights we spent together, I'd wait until after the lights were dimmed to go to the bathroom and wash up. In the morning, before my second snooze alarm went off, I'd get up to "pee" and casually return to bed with my face coated in some of the tinted moisturizer I'd stashed in his cabinet.

During the beginning of our relationship, as my chin became ever more pockmarked, I worried that Charlie's dog might be partially to

blame. For every ounce of Baron the Beagle's adorableness and compan-
ionship, there was about double that in hair. Even going through one
lint roller a week, I was nevertheless finding short white strands on black
leggings I had never worn to Charlie's apartment. And in the wintertime,
Charlie liked to sleep with a heating pad in the shape of an overweight
beagle (even when there was a slightly less furry human option lying right
next to him).

My dermatologist, Dr. K, was unconvinced that sleeping on pillows
covered in dog hair was a factor. Instead, she wanted to know about what
products my new mate was using on his face, which was pretty much
nothing. Charlie didn't even wash with cleanser at night and yet had
perfect skin, which only made my own shame more charged.

Though my face had improved since the vice detox, I still wasn't sure
how confident I felt about going makeup-free in front of Charlie any day
of the week. Wasn't there something to be said for what a polished look
does for your self-worth? If putting on powder every day made me feel
less stressed about the state of my skin, would
I be doing more harm than good by going
without it?

Perhaps in search of a loophole, this was
the question I posed to Dr. Amy Wechsler,
and her answer was a resounding yes: makeup
can do amazing things for your self-esteem,
while stress is a lose-lose.

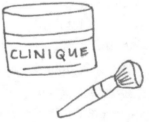

Before she made a career pivot to dermatology, Dr. Wechsler was a
psychiatrist. So when I started to research the impact of anxiety on my
face, her book *The Mind-Beauty Connection: 9 Days to Reverse Stress Aging
and Reveal More Youthful, Beautiful Skin* was the place I started.

Our skin has its own stress response system, she explained. "Just
think about it. When you're happy, your skin glows. If you get frightened,

you turn white as a ghost. What we are thinking and how we are feeling has an outward appearance."

Dr. Wechsler pegs cortisol, the hormone that gets released into the bloodstream when we feel anxiety, as the chief enemy of our skin's health. The inflammation that results causes more nerve fibers to form, which makes already sensitive skin even more so. People who are prone to acne get hit much harder when they're under pressure.

"There was even a study on college campuses that found pimples increase by fifty percent during exams!" she told me.

If the average American has about fifty brief stress spikes a day, I was guessing mine jumped to sixty during that first Makeup-Free Monday. I had cleared my schedule so I could tether myself indoors, using the white lie of an article deadline to bow out of a movie date with Charlie that night. But keeping myself out of sight from others didn't make my own eyes any more forgiving.

Though my imperfections had become less noticeable than the month prior, seeing them completely exposed made my chest tighten every time I caught a glimpse of my patchy skin in the mirror in between baking batches of minimally sweetened granola. And according to Dr. Wechsler, even these minor emotional flare-ups take a toll on the skin's ability to protect you from the outside world.

In one study, researchers tested the skin's stress response by irritating an area of the arm with a piece of tape. After applying and ripping it off a few times, they measured the amount of moisture that seeped out of the affected area. They found that the skin of those who had also been given the added stress of attending a mock job interview afterward had been significantly weakened compared to those who experienced the tape irritation in isolation of any emotional pressures.

"If that's what happens in the lab," said Wechsler, "think about what happens in real life when a fake job interview is the least of your pressures."

Toxic Relationships

With that first makeup-free test behind me until the following week, I shifted my focus to the second most stressful aspect of my green beauty experiment: figuring out what to buy and how much it would cost me.

On a Wednesday afternoon, armed with my iPhone, I began the process of assessing my bathroom landscape. I had downloaded the Environmental Working Group's app, Skin Deep, to see where my current routine fell on their toxicity scale. I'd begin by swapping out the biggest offenders and go from there. Seeing my cabinets with fresh eyes, though, revealed that this task would be easier said than done.

On the bottom shelf was a canvas organizer with twenty assorted lipsticks and glosses, three half-used CoverGirl blushes, and four seldom-used Lancôme eye shadow palettes. On the next shelf, like a chipmunk storing up for winter in the Bahamas, I'd stockpiled Kiehl's entire line of sunscreen (think every size, every SPF) and a good dozen packet samples that had expired in 2009. And the list goes on (and on).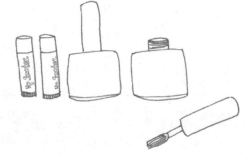

Like other girls desperately fighting their awkward stage, I started my makeup collection in teendom with white eyeliner and other "statement" applications I could use to distract from the three pounds of metal in my mouth. And it expanded even further the summer going into my senior year, when I scored an unpaid internship at a fashion magazine.

Once a season, the beauty editors would put on sale all of the free samples in their possession, most of which had never even been opened, all priced at one dollar. Like a kid in a candy store, I came home that summer with an armload of disturbingly vibrant blue eye shadows and bronzers that were five ethnicities too dark for me. Nonetheless, I held on to my summer peach and very-berry lip glosses for over a decade— until this project helped me realize that those pretty pink face crayons contained multiple parabens associated with breast cancer.

Today, teenagers use even more products than adults—an average of seventeen a day. At the same time, girls are now getting their periods as early as six years old. Researchers are beginning to connect the dots— one study by Mount Sinai School of Medicine discovered a high incidence of endocrine disruptors found in nail polishes and other cosmetics when they examined girls with early-onset puberty. Even small tweaks to your hormone levels can affect the whole motherboard. It made me wonder if my early obsession with metallic nail polish and eye shadow, and the endocrine-disrupting chemicals they housed, had any effect on my thyroid issues later in life.

According to the Skin Deep app, half of my stash ranked as a code red 10 out of 10. The label of my body lotion even recommended I visit a poison control center if I accidentally got any in my mouth.

As with any toxic relationship, though, it was hard to shake my warped sense of attachment. These brands had made me countless promises of beauty and perfection, and whether or not they had kept their word, they had been an armor of protection that had made me feel so much better about my flaws over the years.

Replacing all of these items at once felt too daunting and expensive. So after consulting with several holistic aestheticians, I decided to begin with the products that stayed on my skin the longest: face and body lotion, deodorant, foundation, and other creams. Their second recommendation was that I invest in a natural cleanser, even though it only stays on your face for a few seconds.

That Clean Feeling

"You've been taught to think of oily skin as the worst thing in the world, but that's confusing the issue," wrote Adina Grigore, who started her line of natural products, S.W. Basics, out of her kitchen. "Your skin's oil is important and you shouldn't think of it as the enemy."

Even Dr. Wechsler, who's not necessarily a fan of green products, said that harsh face washes were a problem. "You want your cleanser to get rid of all the dirt but leave your natural oils behind. So many brands leave your skin sort of squeaky-clean. But if you're squeaky-clean, you're *too* clean."

When my skin was at its worst, I'd revert to the Clean & Clear (and under control!) commercials of my adolescence and fiercely wash my face as often as possible. But in removing all the oiliness, I had apparently just been causing more oil to appear as my skin desperately attempted to hydrate and protect itself. As someone with sensitive skin, I was told that I should use a gentle cleanser and wash my face only once a day (at night). After years of scrubbing with acne-fighting micro beads, though, I couldn't quite picture just splashing my face with water in the morning and calling it a day.

"There's this mindset, at least in America, that if something doesn't sting or burn, it's not working," said Dr. Wechsler. "I have to dispel that myth all the time."

This was, indeed, one reason I had dragged my feet for so long to make the switch to naturals. I worried that the new products wouldn't work as effectively. But perhaps it was just that they wouldn't feel or look like what I was used to.

I came across an interesting example of this personal-care psychology in Charles Duhigg's *The Power of Habit: Why We Do What We Do in Life and Business*.

Until famed advertising exec Claude C. Hopkins took on the client

Pepsodent in the early 1900s, there was no market for toothpaste in America. Many credit the success of his campaign as the foundation of our modern tooth-brushing habit. But while instilling a need for Americans to get that "dirty film" off their teeth definitely helped Pepsodent succeed where many toothpaste brands failed, market researchers later discovered one essential difference in the formula itself.

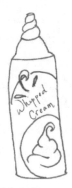

Pepsodent's toothpaste contained chemicals that were mild irritants, which created a tingling feeling on the tongue and gums. The researchers found that when consumers used other brands (and therefore didn't get this tingly sensation), they reported that their mouths didn't feel as clean.

The chemicals didn't make the product work any better. But the tingling convinced people it was doing its job. Today, every mainstream toothpaste brand now contains these ingredients, along with foaming agents such as sodium laureth sulfate, which has been known to cause irritation to the skin, eyes, and lungs, in addition to lather.

It was hard to imagine my face and body washing routine without that whipped-cream-can foam, and all the Herbal Essence–style moans that came with it. But these weren't the things I was after anymore. Knowing that I'd be forgoing arbitrary and unnecessary ingredients mattered more in the long term than simply washing off the day. And that type of clean feeling—both inside and out—seemed like a worthy trade-off.

A Not-So-Natural Woman

Many health-conscious folks look at food labels every day—especially those of us scanning for sugar—but how often do we read the ingredients list when shopping for lotion?

It's something I never thought about before my inaugural trip to the body section of Whole Foods to pick up new face wash and moisturizer. I immediately got sidetracked by all the gleaming bottles and felt my old hoarding impulses kick in as I zeroed in on labels emblazoned with pictures of pitted avocados and pomegranate seeds.

But when I started looking at the backs of the packages, things got confusing. The general ingredients-list rule of thumb for beauty is the same as it is for food: if you can't pronounce it, chances are it's not good for you (with the exception of the word "acai"). The problem, though, is that a lot of natural brands list plant extracts in Latin, and even some of the more natural options had stabilizers sandwiched in between their tea tree oil and organically grown marshmallow. After reading the fifth ingredient, my eyes began to glaze over and made me wish I still drank coffee.

All you need to do is turn on the TV to know that "natural" is now a concept that advertisers have exploited. And unfortunately, as is true for granola bars and canned soup, there are no strict federal standards to restrict the use of the word on cosmetic packaging. Using "natural" and its related terms (along with pictures of avocados) is what clean beauty advocates call "greenwashing."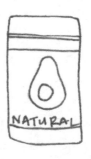

Take Aveda, for example. It was one of the first companies to put plant-based hair-care products on the map in 1978 (ironically, the same year Dan Rather introduced the word "wellness" to mainstream America). When Horst Rechelbacher founded the company, his approach was seen as counterculture, something that would likely recede with the tide of postwar hippies polluting the rhythm of capitalism with their eco tote bags and patchouli oil. Instead, his company grew and Rechelbacher became a powerful advocate for the green movement. His most famous tactic, used at conferences to illustrate his belief that "you shouldn't put anything on your skin that you wouldn't put in your mouth," was to drink his own hair spray.

Today, Aveda is owned by billion-dollar parent company Estée Lauder. And despite using that same green messaging it was so famous for in Rechelbacher's heyday, the ingredients in their hair care products today tell a different story. In addition to the natural extracts listed, including the aforementioned organically grown marshmallow, there were also several parabens and a handful of other chemicals that I definitely couldn't pronounce.

When you start shipping globally, it's hard to scale without adding some sort of stabilizer. But I highly doubted Horst Rechelbacher would want them in his morning smoothie.

If I was going to go fully green, I had to take every single ingredient—Latin or not—into account. The best tactic seemed to be to buy products with as few as possible, like the Dr. Bronner's Organic Virgin Coconut Oil I put in my cart. No need to vet the ingredients list with a fine-tooth comb: there was just one thing on there.

Balancing My Beauty Budget

As a health-focused private chef, I thought of Whole Foods as Mecca. And since I made a pilgrimage there several times a week, I'd developed tactics for not dropping a significant portion of my rent money at the checkout counter. But when the tab for my new products topped $178—more than I would spend to cater a twenty-person cocktail party—I was genuinely taken aback.

The benefits of taking on each of my lifestyle changes in isolation was that I could budget better for them. One reason why the sweeping advice from my endocrinologist and celebrity wellness experts had felt so unattainable was its effect on my financial wellness. So often I had found myself mindlessly throwing money at my health problems at every impulse. For this project, I wanted to commit to spending my dollars in a more thoughtful way by establishing a monthly wellness slush fund.

I put mine around the $150 mark, knowing that I could afford this by eliminating other expenses that didn't fuel my health, like shoes. Some months I might direct it toward acupuncture or blood work, others foot massages or fitness memberships. I wanted to avoid impulse buys and unnecessary doodads, and understood that some months I might have some carryover, while others, like this green beauty experiment, required more up-front investment.

For the women who drop three hundred dollars on a 1-ounce bottle of La Mer Regenerating Serum, the idea of naturals being prohibitive is a joke. But for those of us who buy our basics at CVS, the fear that we'll have to spend more to switch to organic products is real. A small thirty-eight-dollar tube of Dr. Hauschka Foundation, something I planned on wearing six days a week, felt like a very different investment than the twelve-dollar L'Oréal equivalent at the drugstore.

I walked out of Whole Foods poorer, but with an armful of Skin Deep–approved, all-natural products: Evan Healy Blue Chamomile Day Moisturizer and Blue Lavender Cleansing Milk, Dr. Bronner's peppermint body wash, Babo Botanicals SPF 30 Clear Zinc Sunscreen Lotion, Tom's of Maine Lavender Deodorant, the aforementioned foundation, and two jars of coconut oil.

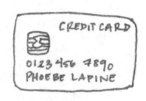

LATER THAT WEEK, I met up with Kerrilynn Pamer and Cindy DiPrima, the founders of CAP Beauty, to discuss why they quit their day jobs to start New York's first boutique for all-natural self-care products. I also hoped they could help me wrap my head around my recent spending spree and explain why the value of green beauty was worth a little extra green.

"The problem is there's a disconnect," mused Kerrilynn about my Whole Foods excursion. "When I'm buying a four-dollar head of broccoli and then I go into the area that has beauty products and see a thirty-dollar moisturizer, I think, 'Well, that's crazy!' But you would never feel that way at Sephora."

Before my market trip, I had done some browsing on natural beauty websites like Spirit Beauty Lounge and Credo Beauty. But it was hard to commit to buying a new, more expensive product online without the option to sniff the jar and smear a little bit of it on the back of my hand to make sure I liked it. Having a comparable experience to what you would get at any boutique or department store was one of the reasons the duo decided to dedicate a brick-and-mortar space to natural beauty. The experience needs to mitigate the price tag by giving you a good idea of what you're buying.

My other related worry was: without synthetic stabilizers, natural beauty products don't last as long. What would that do to my beauty budget?

"Of course a canned peach is going to last longer than a beautiful fresh peach," explained Cindy. "But wouldn't you prefer the fresh one?" In fact, she argued, the shorter shelf life would actually save me money by breaking my beauty overbuying habit. She even had a term for it: "pantry-loading."

Cindy, a former food prop stylist, had heard the term while working on an ad campaign for deli meat. "The director told the recipe developer to avoid any obscure condiments. 'You know,' he said, 'the pantry-loading items.' Meaning the things people randomly buy and never use, like jalapeño chutney and southwestern lamb seasoning blends."

Considering I probably had those two exact items shoved at the back of my kitchen cabinet, it was safe to say that I was a pantry loader.

"If you're putting moisturizer on your face twice a day, there's no reason you need it to last five years."

I agreed with her. But I still wanted my new forty-dollar face cream to get me through at least a few months. The CAP ladies assured me that natural formulas also tend to be more concentrated. Most family-size lotions at the drugstore seem to offer more for less. But it's mostly thanks to the formula's primary ingredient: water. Naturals focus on high-quality oils and botanicals, which last longer without stabilizers if they're not diluted with water. Meaning, less is actually more than you think.

I hoped they were right, and that like that jalapeño chutney, a little blue chamomile moisturizer would indeed go a long way.

Cosmetic Cleanup

I started seeing the benefits of my new natural beauty routine almost immediately, the first being simplicity: instead of having a full arsenal of masks, serums, toners, spot busters, and under-eye whiteners, I'd reduced my daily skin-care routine to just a few essentials.

My lavender cleansing milk worked just as well as, if not better than, my old products, despite the lack of tingly foam, and left my skin feeling soft and lacquered instead of buffed and raw. It was as if someone had turned the houselights on in the outer layer of my skin, and this newfound glow made the minor imperfections—all those healing acne pockmarks—fade into the background.

The coconut oil took a little more getting used to.

It felt strange sticking my hands in a jar that would ordinarily sit on my kitchen counter, and even stranger slathering something I might use to fry an egg all over my legs. But afterward, my calves glistened like they belonged in a Nair commercial (despite the fact that I hadn't shaved them in weeks).

I had less success using it as a hair mask, which left my blond strands looking dark and damp until the following shower—a matter made worse by the fact that I was also experimenting to see if taking a break from shampoo would help the state of my scalp.

Another one of my ongoing beauty woes was dandruff. Now that I had made the connection between my autoimmune issues and the flare-ups that were happening on my face, I was beginning to suspect that the state of my scalp was yet another indication of an internal ecosystem that had gone off the rails. But this was one issue that the vice detox hadn't really cured, which made me think that my hair products might be making matters worse.

The foaming agents in conventional shampoos are surfactants, which act more like a laundry detergent than a soap. They are very effective at removing oil and dirt. But like harsh facial cleansers, this may not always be a good thing. Many people in the curly hair no-poo movement avoid surfactants because natural oils keep their ringlets tight, shiny, and Penny Lane–esque. Other people simply have scalp reactions to these chemicals, which are meant more for hair than skin.

In terms of toxic urgency, my hair products were low on my list. Though the chemicals are often the same as in other products, the contact is limited, and any exposure gets rinsed away within seconds. To keep my beauty budget in check, I had planned on swapping out my shampoo and conditioner once my current bottles ran out.

In the meantime, though, I wanted to heal my scalp. One article suggested the best way to do so would be to go au naturel for a few days, allowing some healthy oils to regenerate and protect my dry skin. Instead, the stark change in hair habits left a buildup of thick, cakey dandruff at my roots. It was too greasy to make my shoulders look like the bottom of a snow globe, but burrowed deep under my fingernails like pie dough every time I went to scratch my temple while reading natural shampoo consumer reports online.

To remedy this, apparently I needed to exfoliate with some help from my kitchen.

So off I went to puree a few large spoonfuls of sour cream with a cubed cucumber. The lactic acid promised to dissolve the buildup of dead skin cells, while the cucumber would comfort and soothe. As I sectioned my hair and slathered the mixture on my exposed scalp with a pastry brush, it felt pleasant and cooling, even if the smell made me feel like I was assembling a crudité platter on my head. After I rinsed thoroughly in the shower, I scratched my scalp and was surprised to find far less gunk.

As the day went on, though, I noticed I had traded one form of dandruff for another; the flakes I had eradicated were replaced with small flecks of cucumber that spun around my wavy tendrils and deposited on my shoulders throughout the evening.

CHARLIE WAS OUT of town for the week, which had given me a safe space to play around with my personal hygiene. And I was grateful for his absence once I experienced some of the other results. My new foundation provided only a chiffon curtain for my blemishes when what I really wanted was a blackout shade, and the scent of my Tom's of Maine lavender deodorant mixed with a little more "eau de moi" than I would have liked. It also left the pits of my white T-shirts tinged yellow.

But these healthy hedonism side effects, though unfortunate, seemed like a small price to pay for feeling better about my new regimen. Once I knew about all their potential hazards, I couldn't look at my old frosted jars of face cream and not see right through them.

With new, clean essentials on board, I knew the next step toward recovery was purging my bathroom of its toxic load.

I felt incredibly wasteful as I filled a garbage bag with half-empty bottles and jars. The plastic heaved and clattered as I dragged it downstairs to the curb. Had I been able to, I probably would have tried to donate my discarded items to Goodwill. But how could I give anyone a bottle of body lotion filled with phthalates that have been proven to cause liver damage and reproductive problems?

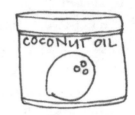

The scariest thing I uncovered was the simple lack of regulation.

There are upward of eighty thousand chemicals in our product pantry today, and only a small fraction of them have been tested for safety. The European Union has banned over eleven hundred ingredients in the last ten years. The United States has failed to regulate even twelve. And that's partly because the laws in place to protect against harmful personal care products haven't been updated since 1938. Manufacturers aren't even required by the Food and Drug Administration to test cosmetics for safety before they hit the market. And if a product is proven harmful, the agency doesn't have the muscle to recall it.

The power is really in consumers' hands to make educated choices. But as I discovered when cleaning out my bathroom and looking on the backs of packages, when brands tout their product as paraben- or sulfate-free, those chemicals are often replaced with new ones that might be equally toxic.

Perhaps, dog hair aside, Charlie's bare-all approach really was the key to the best skin care.

Make Me Up, Before You Go-Go

Switching out my makeup was a whole other psychological beast. The chemical argument was just as strong for these products, but given my attachment to them, it was easier to say the positive emotional effects might trump the negative health ones. To feel like the switch was really worth it, I needed convincing that nontoxic makeup would actually make me prettier. And Kristen Arnett, the founder of the website Green Beauty Team, did exactly that.

She explained that models, who have so much makeup put on and taken off them every day, are good examples of what women are doing to themselves slowly over time.

"I've been a makeup artist for more than a decade. By the time fashion month is over, these poor girls . . . their skin is destroyed," she told me over the phone. "Many of them are teenagers, and they've actually started to develop allergies to mainstream makeup brands. So what that tells me in regard to regular women is: you might not see it today, you might not see it tomorrow, but eventually you're going to see the effects of putting harsh chemicals on your skin."

And with that, I asked if she would give me a natural makeup consultation to finally take the leap.

When I arrived at her apartment, Kristen had her wheelie bags of expertly packed cosmetics unzipped in the living room and ready for rummaging.

We began with a little show-and-tell of my current makeup items. And as I pulled out a crumbling CoverGirl blush with its cracked plastic compact that I'd actually taped shut at the hinge, I started to feel self-conscious.

"This stuff is so weak," Kristen remarked as she brushed some on the back of her hand. "Do you see how faint that mark is? And that's the darkest color in your palette. No wonder you use it up so fast."

Next I handed over my beloved Superpowder, already having separation anxiety as she examined it.

"Isn't Clinique supposed to be hypoallergenic?" I asked hopefully, having embraced blissful ignorance by not searching this item on the Skin Deep app.

Kristen smelled the hand she'd just powdered and wrinkled her nose.

"I highly doubt it," she said. "This stuff is full of fragrance."

She explained that as unregulated as most beauty products are, "parfums" are protected as a trade secret. Brands don't have to disclose any of the ingredients—and there can be over two hundred in any one formula.

This didn't come as a surprise to me. The biggest irony of my green transition was that my first job out of college was in the beauty industry, a professional posting that only added a hundred more products to my pantry. And in this former life, one of my roles was developing women's fragrances.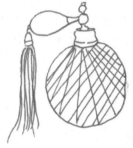

During meetings, the requisite French alpha male in charge would ask, "Who has clean skin?" And being the lone woman not already wearing one of the company's signature scents, I would be volunteered as tribute. This entailed having my wrists sprayed with all the prototypes under review, then walking around the room so that the other French alpha males could sniff their way up my forearms. For most of that year, I left the office with a headache, smelling and feeling like a baby prostitute. I didn't need to look at the internal ingredients lists on those samples to know that the chemicals in them didn't agree with my body.

"There are some pretty credible studies that show that when a man is sprayed with synthetic cologne, within three minutes his sperm count drops thirty-three percent," Kristen chimed in, which made me think that perhaps for women over the age of sixteen, Axe Body Spray acts as a natural birth control in more ways than just as a repellent.

After she'd washed her hands of my contaminated cosmetics, Kristen showed me the basics of an everyday makeup routine for adult women. By the time she finished, I'd written down seven products and three brushes—including a W3LL People Blush, Jane Iredale Eye Pencil, Abbey St Clare Concealer, and various Alima Pure powders—I needed to purchase in order to achieve my new "after" look.

"It takes a lot more finesse to get a subtle, natural glow than it does to look like a corpse bride on Halloween," she added.

I wanted to be a good student and go buy all of my new tools. But after seeing they would set me back another two hundred dollars, I decided to stick with just the essentials I would use every day and replace some of the rest over time.

Green or otherwise, I didn't want to hoard again in the name of perfection.

The Sweet Spot

Because I mostly worked from home, if I wanted to hide my makeup-free face, I could do so by never leaving the house. But once I finally got up the courage to go out in public, I realized that being around other people didn't make me any more self-conscious than I already was cooped up by myself. What I saw staring back at me through my thick lens of self-criticism during those first few makeup-free Monday mornings was what my preteen idol Cher Horowitz would have called a full-on Monet:

"Fine from far away, but up close, a big old mess." And those distortions only got harsher the more time I had to dwell on them.

The experiment had a big long-term benefit, though.

The less makeup I wore, the more I got used to my bare face, and the less I seemed to mind the lack of coverage from my new sheer foundation. It helped break my dependency on mindless makeup. Between the vice detox, giving my face an occasional breather from brushes, sponges, and creams, and switching my products to naturals, my skin improved so much over the course of two months that I didn't care as much about concealing it.

With my new scaled-down routine firmly established, I finally got the courage to talk to Charlie about my skin shame and the previous, devious tactics I used to hide it. Always a calm and nonchalant sounding board for my worries, he shrugged off the revelation.

"Your face was never that bad," he told me.

"That's because I wore makeup all the time!"

To prove my point, I pulled up one of the detox selfies on my phone, an image that still made me cringe. Charlie stared at it for a minute, his ample brows furrowed. As his eyes detailed the whitehead above my lip and the raw red patches around my mouth, I felt a little pang of that old anxiety.

He looked up and took in the comparison.

"Well," he said, his forearm curling around to rest on the back of my neck. "I must have been so crazy about you that I never really noticed."

IT WAS CLEAR that the cost of going green paid in the long term.

By far the most helpful aspect of having

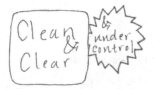

Kristen by my side was having her match my skin tone on the first try. Many natural brands, like Alima Pure, offer small sample sizes you can mail-order to test on your skin. But it's still much easier to have an expert choose for you as you might at a department store counter. Boutiques like CAP Beauty are beginning to crop up in bigger cities. And big retailers like Target and Walmart are catching up to the need for naturals elsewhere. Until their selection grows, though, Whole Foods is still probably the most accessible place to start your green beauty transition in person.

The best way around money is often time. By swapping my products over a longer period, I could have avoided blowing my monthly wellness budget. Upgrading most of my skin care at once allowed me to see a more immediate impact, but it came at a higher up-front cost.

There were still a few items from my old product pantry that I held on to: mascaras, eye shadows, lipsticks—the things I only wore on special occasions. Reducing my everyday toxins made me less stressed out about the times I used hotel shampoo or reverted back to these old products in the name of fun. Like the occasional slice of gluten-free cake, I didn't want to worry about indulging in my favorite neon pink statement lip or overspending to replace all of the colors in my collection.

As time went on, I came to value the way natural products made my skin feel more than any synthetic functionality.

Sometimes I'd revert back to my old powder compact when I was in a rush or needed something to pop in my purse for touch-ups. But now when I looked at my even, perfectly powdered face, it didn't look the same. I didn't see flawless coverage. I just saw makeup.

"Waterproof mascara performs so well *because* it has synthetic, waterproof ingredients," says Jessa Blades, a green makeup artist and the founder of Blades Natural Beauty. "If you're getting married, or you're a swimsuit model jumping in and out of a pool, those ingredients are helpful and important. But for the average person who has the ability to touch up in the office bathroom if she needs to, nontoxic products are great for everyday use. We just have to be realistic with our expectations. As of right now, natural lipsticks aren't going to come in as many colors, cost as little, be as easy to find, or last up to twenty-four hours. But do we really need them to?"

THOUGH I LOVED my new clean routine, one of my biggest realizations of my green beauty transition was that, like pills, I couldn't rely on products alone to fight my skin's battles for me. Most aestheticians, dermatologists, and even makers of the natural beauty lines I bought agreed that what we put on our skin can only go so far.

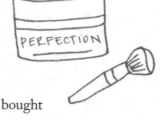

When I woke up wan from drinking one more glass of wine than I should have, a little blue chamomile moisturizer could only breathe so much light back into my complexion. Rinsing my face gently with lavender cleansing milk would only do so much for preventing breakouts. The evidence of a gluten-free chocolate chip cookie I had indulged in at a potluck party was written all over my chin the next morning. Paying attention to how my vices, even in moderation, played out over my face was even more reason to keep making sure that I only indulged in treats when they truly felt like treats, on occasions that actually were special.

Because what we feed ourselves does so much more for our outward-facing health than any potion ever could. And I knew that even after my detox there was still a lot more work to be done on that front.

Healthy Hedonist Natural Beauty Tips

Switching to naturals doesn't need to be an expensive or stressful process. You can make the transition slowly, swapping products as they run out. And you can choose the sweet spot where that transition ends.

1. *Keep a product journal.* Record everything you come into contact with, including mouthwash and hand soap, what time you use what, and any noticeable changes in your skin. This is something people often do for food but rarely for their skin-care products. Adina Grigore recommends the practice in her fabulous book *Skin Cleanse: The Simple, All-Natural Program for Clear, Calm, Happy Skin*, as a way to (1) see how many items you're actually using, and (2) notice the problem products.

2. *Go cold turkey for twenty-four hours.* Give all of your products a rest for one day. If the list of chemicals in your bathroom isn't reason enough to pare down your routine, then perhaps simply seeing the results of what your skin can do on its own might convince you to cut back on the items you use (and the number of ingredients in them) going forward.

3. *Check databases for red flags.* Do a quick cross-reference of your favorite products on the Think Dirty app or the Environmental Working Group's app, Skin Deep. If it's a level 4 or 5, it's probably not necessary to throw it away immediately. But a code red 10 out of 10? Consider a natural replacement pronto.

4. *Replace the items that stay on your body the longest first.* Exposure does matter when it comes to toxic chemicals. Start your

transition with lotions, creams, and any everyday items that either absorb into your skin or that you wear all day long.

5. *Take off your makeup at night!* Don't skip this step. It could be a huge cause of your breakouts, regardless of what types of products you're using. Nighttime is when your skin detoxes, so make sure it's clean enough to let your pores breathe. A cotton swab with olive, coconut, or avocado oil works great as a natural eye makeup remover.

6. *Put fragrance on your clothes, not your skin.* If you can't part with your signature scent, try to avoid getting it on your skin where it gets absorbed into your bloodstream. Spray it on what you're wearing instead.

7. *Have a dedicated face towel.* Drying your face with a clean cloth will remove the risk of inadvertently rubbing irritating products like hand soap, deodorant, or your partner's aftershave on your face. Holistic aesthetician Nichola Weir of Pacific Touch NYC recommends using something particularly soft, like a baby towel, if you have sensitive skin. Gently dab your face dry instead of wiping it. Also, avoid using gym towels since those tend to be rough and treated with intense cleaning chemicals. Speaking of which, consider switching to natural detergent.

8. *Wash your makeup brushes.* You use these on your face every day and they can be as much of a magnet for dust, bacteria, and dirt as anything else in your home. If you find that your makeup routine is irritating your skin, try cleaning your brushes first with gentle, unscented castile soup. Tack this chore onto Makeup-Free Monday and you can give your brushes a cleaning while your face is taking a break from them.

9. *Wear sunscreen, period.* Most natural sunscreens contain zinc oxide, and a downside is that they never completely rub in. Though vampire-in-training might not be your preferred look, broad-spectrum mineral sunscreens are the safest option since they don't seep into your skin, are stable in sunlight, and offer UVA protection. Babo Botanicals Clear Zinc Lotion is one that rubs in nicely. But it's better to wear a conventional alternative than nothing.

10. *Banish body odor the natural way.* Preventing our bodies from sweating is not good for our overall health. Skin flora, the natural bacteria under your arms, helps keep you safe by literally eating the toxins in your sweat. Natural deodorants, like Blissoma Scentless Stick or Soapwalla Deodorant Cream, absorb the odor instead of killing your flora with harsh chemicals that leach into your breast ducts. And they actually work.

For a full list of the products in my everyday makeup bag and shower caddy and where to buy them, see Appendix B (page 347).

SWEET AND SPICY PEPITA-CASHEW SNACK MIX

Makes 2¹/₂ cups

Instead of grabbing a sugary energy bar or a bag of greasy potato chips for an on-the-go snack, pack a baggie of this sweet and spicy nut-and-seed mix. Thanks to the pumpkin seeds, cashews, and coconut, it's perfect for promoting skin renewal, protecting against sun damage, and adding a healthy glow that's especially hard to come by when you're traveling.

....

1 cup raw unsalted pumpkin seeds (pepitas)

1 cup raw unsalted cashews

¹/₄ cup finely shredded unsweetened coconut

¹/₄ teaspoon Madras curry powder

¹/₄ teaspoon garam masala

¹/₄ teaspoon cayenne pepper

¹/₂ teaspoon coarse sea salt

2 tablespoons honey

1 large egg white

1. Position a rack in the center of the oven and preheat the oven to 350°F. Line a rimmed baking sheet with parchment paper.

2. In a large mixing bowl, combine the pumpkin seeds, cashews, coconut, curry powder, garam masala, cayenne, and salt. Add the honey and egg white and stir until very well combined. Arrange the mixture in an even layer on the prepared baking sheet, doing your best to separate any clumps.

3. Bake for 20 to 25 minutes, stirring to redistribute the nut mixture every 5 to 10 minutes, until browned and crunchy.

4. Remove from the oven and allow the snack mix to cool completely on the pan. Break up any remaining clusters with your hands and store in an airtight container for nibbling throughout the week.

HEALTHY HEDONIST TIPS

One particularly powerful skin food is zinc, which helps with cell regrowth of the outer layers. Pumpkin seeds are a really great source, and they help release tryptophan, so having some before bed can help with your beauty sleep too. You can also find zinc in whole grains and seafood. If snacking on a dozen oysters isn't your thing, keep this recipe on hand.

MARKET SWAPS

If you want to make this mixture vegan, simply omit the egg and swap maple syrup for the honey. The end result might be a little stickier, but that just makes the snack mix more finger-licking good, right? You can also substitute a variety of nuts and seeds—especially other skin-friendly ones such as sunflower or sesame seeds, pecans or pine nuts—and get creative with the seasonings. Use chili powder and cinnamon (instead of curry and garam masala) for a Mexican twist.

RAW GINGERBREAD COOKIE BEAUTY BALLS

Makes 2 dozen balls

Raw energy balls (the artist formerly known as vegan truffles) have swept the food and wellness blogosphere in recent years. And who am I not to join the party? This version is one of my favorites. They taste like a ginger cookie but are loaded with fiber, antioxidants, and healthy fats thanks to skin superstars like sesame seeds, almond butter, and flax meal. Store them in the fridge for anytime you need a sweet bite that won't throw your blood sugar into turmoil.

....

3/4 cup almond butter

1/4 cup sesame seeds

1 cup gluten-free rolled oats

1/2 cup finely shredded unsweetened coconut

1/2 cup ground flaxseed meal

1 teaspoon ground cinnamon

1/2 teaspoon ground ginger

1/4 teaspoon ground cloves

1/4 teaspoon sea salt

1/4 cup maple syrup

1. Combine all of the ingredients in a large mixing bowl; stir until the mixture is incorporated and sticky. Place the bowl in the refrigerator for 10 minutes, or until firm.

2. With damp hands, take 1 tablespoon of dough and shape it into a compact 1-inch ball and place it on a plate. (Keep a bowl of water by your side, since the mixture is easier to handle with damp hands.) Repeat with

the remaining batter. Chill the balls until ready to serve, or up to 2 weeks, or in the freezer until you remember they're in there.

HEALTHY HEDONIST TIPS

What you've been told about chocolate causing pimples is a myth. It's really the sugar! (Duh.) The hedonist in me feels compelled to say that if you added ½ cup of dark chocolate chips, these bites wouldn't taste terrible. Choose bittersweet (60 percent cacao or higher), or go the healthy route and just add cacao nibs.

MARKET SWAPS

Trade the spices for a few teaspoons of cocoa powder to make these full-fledged raw chocolate "cookies." You can also substitute or add maca powder, which helps fine-tune TRH and TSH messages that impact how many hormones the thyroid produces and is packed with B vitamins, which thyroid peeps tend to be deficient in. This recipe uses a modest amount of maple syrup, which not only gives the balls their requisite sweetness but also holds them together. Raw honey is a great option, as are ⅓ cup chopped Medjool dates. Just puree them in the bowl of a food processor along with the almond butter and add the resulting paste to the bowl.

GUT GUILT

EATING WITHOUT ABANDON

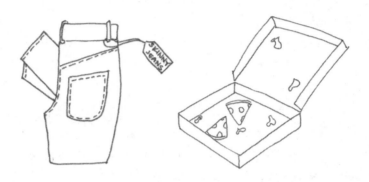

On anti-inflammatory dieting, without fearing food.

ood was the lifestyle area I had changed the most, but despite my oc-
cupation (and partially because of it), my diet was still what caused me
the most angst and confusion.

During my postcollege years, when I let my Hashimoto's run amok, I
started dropping pounds at a rapid rate. After embracing my undergrad
experience as one big all-you-can-eat buffet, along with the late-night
pizza and pounds that came with it, losing weight felt good, no matter
how bad my body felt otherwise.

Skinny was a great perk that came at the price of a lot of misery. If my
stomach hadn't stopped behaving—and if I hadn't had the flu all the
time and felt exhausted even on the days when I didn't—I might have
continued to embrace this weird health loophole of eating whatever I
wanted while wasting away. Eventually, though, when the intestinal pain

got too intense and I started to look like Christian Bale's body double in *The Machinist*, I decided to see a doctor.

At the behest of my homeopathic-minded mother, I sought out someone who practiced functional medicine, an integrative approach to the underlying cause of illness. He did blood work to test for food allergies and put me on an elimination diet to see if there was something that didn't agree with my system. For two weeks, I cut out soy, corn, dairy, sugar, and wheat. And once that agony came to a close, with results in hand, it was clear that I had a serious gluten sensitivity.

The news devastated me. As much as having to lie in the fetal position after every meal was an occupational hazard, being an aspiring chef and food writer with allergies was an even more formidable prospect (I'd been crossing my fingers for tapeworm). The diagnosis came precisely one week before my first cookbook hit stores, and I had trouble finding the irony in the situation as I slaved over batches of chocolate chip cookies for the launch party without being able to so much as lick the spatula. Worse, I was setting off to promote a book that contained one hundred recipes, half of which I could no longer eat.

Once I made it through the five stages of grief and got used to my new dietary restrictions, it was clear that going off gluten was a big step in the right direction. I gained some weight back. As I did, the color returned to my cheeks and my eyes took down their vacancy sign. It made me realize that being skinny didn't necessarily mean being healthy, and being healthy was far more important.

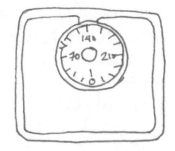

And yet, I still didn't understand why I had been losing so much weight in the first place. An underactive thyroid, which is the main symptom of Hashimoto's thyroiditis, typically makes people put on pounds. Why had my gluten sensitivity caused me to do the opposite?

This, along with how my gluten and autoimmune issues were connected, was never explained to me during those doctor's visits when I was twenty-five. And as a result, I hadn't been as careful on the gluten-free front as I should have been—even during the first few months of my wellness project.

It would have been much easier to get on board if I had celiac disease, where the damage is cut and dry. For celiac sufferers, a bite of gluten causes antibodies to attack the villi of your small intestines. Even the smallest cross-contamination—a few bread crumbs from an artisanal grilled cheese on the deli counter—can set off a reaction. But gluten "sensitivity"? That didn't sound threatening enough to keep me from licking frosting off the tops of wedding cakes.

Thanks to Gloria the Healer's pills, I was finally about to connect all of the dots on the diet front and get the motivation I needed to up the ante: for the next month, I was going to fully commit to anti-inflammatory eating.

I'd take a break from dairy and refined grains, and finally get serious about gluten. No more picking croutons out of Caesar salad, no more using just a few maki rolls' worth of soy sauce at a sushi restaurant. And no more turning a blind eye when my French fries were clearly contaminated with a thin crust of flour from the fryer. (Not to mention those crumb-covered bites of cake frosting.)

The true challenge would be figuring out how to still nurture my love of food within this more restrictive framework. Because if there's one diet rule I'd already learned the hard way, it's that if you're obsessing over what you're eating all the time, no amount of kale salad can make you healthy.

Calling Off the Troops

The vice detox had had a nice halo effect on my eating habits.

I may have been drinking again, but being more aware of the sugar content in everyday packaged foods made me better about passing them up. I was still making my own breakfast (most of the time), and still attempting to forgo unnecessary French desserts. But despite these changes, that initial surge of energy I felt during the monthlong reboot had since worn off—so much so that I was tempted to start drinking more caffeine again to offset my general mental and physical droopiness.

Luckily, one round of blood work later I had an answer: my thyroid antibodies were off the charts. A "normal" TPOAb (thyroid peroxidase antibody) result is somewhere below 30. Mine was at 2,000.

I had been so good about detoxing my life—getting off coffee, limiting added sugar, ridding my skin care of endocrine disruptors, things that should have thrown my thyroid fewer curveballs. Why was this happening now?

When I arrived at my acupuncturist Heidi's office, she had her laptop open in the treatment room with a tab open for each of the supplements Gloria the Healer had given me.

"Mystery solved," she said in a sarcastically cheerful tone. "Wheat germ. You were basically eating three thousand milligrams of gluten a day."

I looked at her in disbelief. And then my eyebrows knitted together into full-on fury. Heidi just gave me a knowing nod.

"I see a lot of patients who've been put on 'natural' pills as a result of muscle testing, or because they read somewhere that it was good for them. You can muscle test till the cows come home, but you've gotta back up the woo-woo. It's about knowing the person, and matching the right remedy to the right situation. That's not something you can pick up off the Internet or over a weekend course."

"I stopped taking those pills months ago, though," I replied, defeated. "Shouldn't they be out of my system by now?"

"Autoimmune issues are tricky," Heidi responded, as she fixed me a cup of calming ginger tea. "Once you have a flare-up, it can be hard to call off the troops.

"Think about it this way," she continued. "You're at a bar, and suddenly someone insults one of your drunk, hot-blooded guy friends. He starts throwing punches left and right, and soon enough, he accidentally hits you in the face. That's autoimmune: when your body can't tell the difference between friend and enemy anymore. Because the gluten protein looks a lot like the thyroid protein, your body has a particularly hard time telling the difference."

A lightbulb went off in my foggy, immunocompromised brain. Where was this bar fight analogy when I was twenty-five?

I finally understood everything that had been staring me in the face for years: leaving my thyroid disease untreated for so long had caused an antibody brawl inside 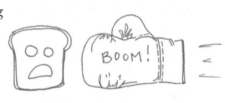 my body, punching even the innocent bystanders, like gluten, who happened to have the same haircut. In the fog of war, my organs struggled to process and absorb nutrients. And the pounds fell off as my body started to dip into its emergency reserves.

By going off gluten four years ago, I had gotten rid of some of the perceived enemies; clearing out the bar had helped my punch-happy immune system take a chill pill. But the problem with living with autoimmune disease—even when you're on medication—is that *anything* can set your body off again. Gluten doesn't just fuel the fight. It can be the dick who starts the whole thing in the first place.

A few weeks of Gloria's wheat germ pills and I had unknowingly provoked another rumble that was still raging on.

Fanning the Flames of Inflammation

There's been a lot of chatter in the media about non-celiac gluten sensitivity and why it's exploded in the last five years.

Contrary to what many believe, GMO white flour has not been approved for sale anywhere in the world. But wheat has been hybridized over the years to withstand increased levels of pesticides. Bread is also made very differently than it was a century ago, with the starkest change being the rise time. A higher percentage of gluten allows factories to develop the elasticity in bread much faster—from twenty-four hours to a mere twenty minutes—through a creepy stabilizing ingredient called vital wheat gluten, which is now added to the majority of processed baked goods.

People may be wary of the validity of gluten sensitivity as it rises at epidemic rates. Many believe that understanding how our food production has changed over the last quarter century is at the helm. But could it also be mimicking the rise of autoimmune disorders in general? How many people are experiencing these misfires as a result of an immune system that has already gone off the rails?

It's estimated that over fifty million Americans suffer from autoimmunity, which includes conditions such as lupus, multiple sclerosis, type 1 diabetes, and rheumatoid arthritis. About 75 percent of all diagnosed are female, which makes it one of the leading causes of death among young and middle-aged women.

There are two opposing sides of the argument as to why this category of illness is on the rise. The hygiene hypothesis says that our systems have become lazy due to an overly clean, man-made world; too much energy spent sterilizing Linus's blanket, and not enough time rolling around in the dirt like Pig Pen. Others say that our immune responses have gone haywire because of unprecedented levels of toxins in our day-to-day lives.

It's hard to know exactly which is the case. But both sides agree that we would all be better off living in the woods without a backpack full of Purell.

Most autoimmune conditions are more alike than they are different, says Dr. Susan Blum, author of *The Immune System Recovery Plan: A Doctor's 4-Step Program to Treat Autoimmune Disease*. And the common thread in all of these internal bar fights is the side effect of inflammation. This is your body's normal response to infection or injury. But if the process goes on for too long or gets out of control, these inflammatory chemicals can interfere with the normal function of your cells and cause tissue damage.

Recently, a lot of professionals have mounted medical soapboxes to speak out against this condition. Among the loudest is Dr. David Perlmutter, a neurologist and the author of *Grain Brain: The Surprising Truth About Wheat, Carbs, and Sugar—Your Brain's Silent Killers*, one of the books that sparked so much gluten hysteria in the first place. In it, Perlmutter points his finger at carbohydrates as our main source of bodily inflammation and, therefore, the cornerstone of all major degenerative conditions, including Alzheimer's, heart disease, and some cancers. It's a pretty extreme argument, one that turns my internal food conversation into a circus of fear every time I eat a bite of brown rice.

"When a person advocates radical change on the order of eliminating one of the three macronutrient groups from our diets, the burden of proof should be enormous," writes the journalist James Hamblin, who profiled

Perlmutter in *The Atlantic*. "To think that every time you eat any kind of carb or gluten, you are putting your mental health and cognitive faculties at risk is, to me, less empowering than paralyzing."

Eat the Rainbow

This paralysis was a familiar feeling—one that I had experienced while listening to the extremist dietary protocol of my endocrinologist, and one I was beginning to get pangs of as I sat at my desk nursing a bowl of salad greens. I had decided to take on a month of anti-inflammatory eating, but being partially unsure of what should be included as part of my new protocol, I had played it safe and stuck with the inarguable power of kale.

Only, as I researched best practices, even my favorite superfood was subject to contradictory speculations.

When I cross-referenced the prevailing anti-inflammatory diets, the no-no foods listed on my yellow legal pad included the trio from my vice detox—alcohol, caffeine, and sugar—along with the big eight allergens: dairy, wheat, eggs, tree nuts, peanuts, shellfish, fish, and soy. Some recommend no seeds, beans, legumes, or grains of any kind. Many only advocate animal protein if it's wild, grass-fed, free-range, or organic. And others said no animal protein at all. Add nightshade vegetables (tomatoes, peppers, potatoes, and eggplant) and cruciferous vegetables (broccoli, cabbage, Brussels sprouts, and, yes, kale) for thyroid sufferers and it starts to feel like all that's left are organic blueberries not flown in from Chile.

It took me years to get on board with my life sans gluten and not want to jump off a building every time there was fresh tagliatelle on a menu. Did I now have to worry about arsenic in rice? Was I really not allowed to eat quinoa unless it had soaked overnight, lest it ferment in my gut? Hadn't this carboholic suffered enough?!

I had already tried weeding out a lot of these items during my first elimination diet years prior, and again after my first session with my endocrinologist Dr. A. The approach might be good for identifying your food triggers, or healing a leaky gut, but as a lifestyle it was too restrictive for me. As dogged as I wanted to be about fighting my inflammation, this project was about finding balance through baby steps. I knew I could never give up all carbs, and taking vegetables with so many beneficial nutrients out of the mix because they contain goitrogens, which can interfere with the thyroid's production of key hormones, just felt beside the point.

I decided to ask my health mentor, Heidi, what food rules she lived by to keep her Hashimoto's at bay. The solution she offered was simple: if you want to follow an anti-inflammatory "diet" without demonizing whole food groups like they're last season's boot-cut jeans, just try to eat according to color.

"Intense hues in fruits and vegetables usually indicate a high level of antioxidants, which limit inflammation," she explained. "Plus steering clear of members of anything in the beige family will help you weed out dairy, bleached carbs, and other processed things that agitate the gut."

These changes seemed doable: orange sweet potatoes over regular spuds, black or brown rice over white, and enough fresh fruit and veggies to make my dinner the most colorful, beautiful plate it could be.

Hopefully, this more moderate approach would be enough to offset the damage Gloria's pills had caused. I'd keep some gluten-free whole grains—oats, brown rice, millet, and quinoa—but steer clear of refined white flours (even gluten-free ones). I'd also try to eliminate dairy, soy, and corn products, which, despite the vibrant yellow or blue hues, are often highly processed and made from GMO seeds.

And lastly, I knew that these modifications would be irrelevant if

I didn't become more vigilant about gluten. Understanding the impact of my small slipups and the wars they were causing in my intestines made me want to do better—not out of guilt or fear but out of sympathy for my body.

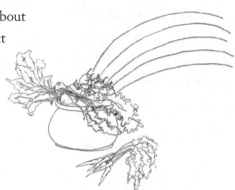

Trial by Tabbouleh Fire

The initial six months of any relationship is a constant parade of firsts. And meeting the parents ranks high as one of the more anxiety-producing ones, right up there with the highly anticipated "I love you" and the dreaded first instance of gas passed in a confined space.

Luckily, I had gotten at least one of these milestones out of the way before Charlie and I had even started dating—that Fourth of July weekend at his mother's house in Rhode Island. But I still had yet to meet his father.

Charlie's relationship with Charlie Sr. had been complicated since his parents' split in his midtwenties. I was beginning to wonder if I'd ever be introduced at all when I got a last-minute text asking if I was free to dine at his dad's apartment the following evening.

It took about six outfit trials before I was ready to walk out the door in the right conservative blend of schoolmarm chic. And as I sat in bumper-to-bumper traffic in midtown, sweating profusely, I began to regret the silk crepe blouse I'd chosen.

When I arrived at the Upper East Side apartment, Charlie's stepmother was the one who answered the door.

"You must be Phoebe," Mrs. M said with a warm smile. "Welcome."

I trailed her perfectly pinned chignon into the open kitchen, where Charlie Jr. was perched at the island with a glass of white wine in his hand. Reluctantly, I handed him my coat, being sure to keep my arms tucked tightly by my sides in order to cover the dark rings of sweat that had formed under them.

"You'll have to excuse my timing—I've been running around all day," said Mrs. M, sweeping a few stray garlic skins from the cutting board. "I hope you don't mind if I put you to work."

My stomach sank when I saw the container of store-bought tabbouleh sitting on the counter. The first few days of my anti-inflammatory eating had been uneventful and easy, mainly because I was the one in charge of my meals. Though I was stressing about keeping up with the conversation at the dinner table without sounding like an uncultured plebe, I felt equally anxious about what would be on the table itself. I tried to catch Charlie's eye as I went about spooning the Middle Eastern salad onto plates, and topping it with slices of smoked salmon, per Mrs. M's instructions. Charlie just stared back at me with wide-eyed confusion, perhaps not realizing that the small beige grains nestled among tomatoes and herbs were bulgur wheat.

"Didn't you warn her?" I whispered under my breath on the way to the dining room.

"I did! Or I thought I did . . ." he replied. "Just tell her—"

Before I could utter the words "No, *you* tell her," my frown turned upside down as Charlie Sr. entered the room and we sat down to supper.

I was grateful to be the one doing most of the talking, to distract from the fact that I was doing none of the eating. My cutlery surveyed the top of the salmon, as I tried to simultaneously cut and scrape. But the specks of bulgur clung to the fish with the ferocity of fine sand on wet feet. It was impossible to avoid.

"All done?" Mrs. M asked before clearing my barely touched plate.

My fear of offending or being labeled as high maintenance seemed to be the inevitable conclusion of this dinner. Charlie reassured me otherwise on the cab ride home, but my stomach churned under the weight of wheat and failed first impressions—the perfect storm of gut guilt.

The next day, I nursed my bloated belly with some warm lemon water and tried not to picture my cowering thyroid, waiting for my immune system to take its next swing of the piñata bat.

Gluten-Freedom

During my first few years off gluten, I was much less concerned with being poisoned by a few stray grains than I was with being hungry.

I didn't fear overeating as much as I feared not eating at all.

Many would argue that this was a positive progression, especially for someone who was once bound by the same scooped-out-bagel shackles that many high school girls wear for fear of gaining weight. I wasn't fanatically recording what I ate or stepping on a scale every morning to see if the banana with peanut butter from my after-school snack made me "fat." Instead, cutting out a food group in my midtwenties had actually helped me make peace with putting on a few more pounds in the name of health.

Only, the pendulum may have swung too far in the other direction.

As I paid more attention to my habits during the week that followed the tabbouleh incident, I realized I had developed a scarcity mindset around my restrictions. When I traveled through gluten-free food deserts, I always did so with a loaf of bread in my carry-on, wedged between my iPad and pink fleece airplane socks, leaving a stream of confused airport Quiznos managers in my wake.

After years of this hassle, finding gluten-free bread on a menu still felt like a novelty—a gift from the dietarily challenged gods. And who was I to defy them by not ordering a sandwich?

I wasn't keeping a food journal, but if I had been, I might have noticed how often I ate a gluten-free pizza, muffin, or other carby treat because it felt like a rare opportunity that had to be taken advantage of rather than a staple that now existed on every other block of Manhattan. I wasn't deluding myself into thinking gluten-free bread was that much healthier than regular bread. But I had, it turns out, been deluding myself that I wasn't eating a whole loaf of it every week.

During the first leg of my anti-inflammatory eating challenge, I felt surprisingly lost.

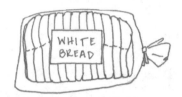

I wholeheartedly believed in the concept of food as medicine, yet my project was already showing me that I wasn't always practicing it on myself. I hadn't thought sugar was a problem until I experienced what happened when it was taken away. Now I was seeing how often my other food vices—mainly, processed simple carbs—had been folded into every meal. It was a wake-up call to realize the percentage of my plate that had been covered by quinoa pasta, millet toast, white rice, and corn tortillas—even if they were also accompanied by a few colors from the vegetable rainbow.

The first week of the experiment, I ate mostly salads for lunch, which felt much less satisfying than my usual avocado toast, veggie burger, or maki combo B. Knowing that consuming the same foods every day, even if it was a bowl of leafy greens, was not necessarily good for me either, I tried to instead come up with a food version of a capsule wardrobe—daily things I could always turn to without overthinking the components: a cup of lentil soup or turkey chili; a plate of grain-free meatballs or rotisserie chicken with roasted vegetables.

Sourcing these options during the day, on my own time, was easy—especially in a city where they could be delivered to my doorstep within minutes. At restaurants, though, I kept feeling like I was stuck in a Nora Ephron scene ordering for Sally Albright.

Meat in the Middle

A few weeks after the tabbouleh incident, I found myself at a Mexican taqueria with some of Charlie's friends, once more being forced into flexibility. Though I remembered to bring my own taro and beet chips (vibrant!) to use as a vehicle for guacamole, I still labored over the menu. Did I get a salad—likely an anemic bed of iceberg lettuce—or hold up the entire ordering process by asking the server ten questions about how the fish entrée was prepared, followed by five modification requests?

Instead, in the outer-body throes of anxiety, I heard a voice that sounded a lot like my own order the carnitas plate.

For the rest of dinner, I alternated between eating around the white rice it came with, and justifying to myself that the fibrous black beans offset the hulled, bleached grains when I snuck a taste. Had I not panic-ordered, I might have had the foresight to ask for no grains or tortillas, which arrived in a wicker basket topped with a miniature sombrero. But seeing as I was already the weirdo who brought her own chips to dinner and wasn't partaking in the shared pitcher of margaritas or queso fundido appetizer, I probably would have just relied on willpower anyway rather than call attention to myself.

Unfortunately, moderation is a lot easier when you set yourself up for success. And less so when the foods you're avoiding are sitting right on your plate. Once the entirety of my pile of matted pork shavings had disappeared, and my tequila on the rocks had sunk in, it was only natural to help myself to a few more unrestrained bites of rice to soak up the alcohol sloshing around in my stomach.

On nights like these—when I ordered an entrée in the name of not being the girl feasting on a side salad— I realized, like those Paleo CrossFitters crushing beef jerky at snack time, the absence of refined grains usually meant more meat.

A rare steak and fillet of salmon get a thumbs-up according to the vibrancy model. I just wasn't sure I was doing my inflammation any favors by eating so much of them. Despite the carb-free, high-protein trends, the majority of scientific studies lean toward the idea that we would all benefit from eating fewer animals. One of the most glaring commonalities across Blue Zone populations—communities with the world's highest percentage of centenarians—was the lack of red meat in their diets. Even seafood was a few-times-per-week treat.

Though animals may be a central part of a "primal diet," the majority of the ones eaten today are much more toxic and inflammatory than what our hunter-gatherer ancestors were accustomed to.

As the world grapples with widespread hunger, 160 countries have felt the need to ban meat produced in the United States to protect their citizens. This is largely due to the drug ractopamine, which keeps animals lean. In humans, however, the substance acts as a stress hormone, raising many red flags for health concerns, particularly among young children. Even mainland China, a country not widely lauded for responsible food safety measures, has banned the drug in feed.

The hormones used in livestock are particularly worrisome for those of us dealing with thyroid issues. Feed additives make their way into our bodies through the vessels we consume and can be just as harmful to our delicate hormonal balance as the endocrine-disrupting body lotion we ingest through our skin.

While a few more plates of sashimi or
shrimp scampi seems like a logical
solution, modern seafood poses
an even more nuanced problem.

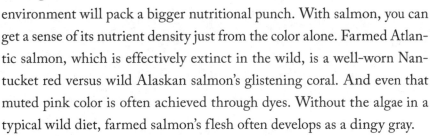

Many nutritionists and
physicians say to go wild.
Like grass-fed cows, fish
feeding in their natural ocean
environment will pack a bigger nutritional punch. With salmon, you can
get a sense of its nutrient density just from the color alone. Farmed Atlantic salmon, which is effectively extinct in the wild, is a well-worn Nan-
tucket red versus wild Alaskan salmon's glistening coral. And even that
muted pink color is often achieved through dyes. Without the algae in a
typical wild diet, farmed salmon's flesh often develops as a dingy gray.

But there are other things to consider besides vibrancy.

One of the most well-studied toxins in relation to autoimmune
disease is mercury, which occurs at high levels in larger wild fish such
as swordfish, marlin, and your favorite garnet sushi-grade tuna. For
Hashimoto's sufferers, these heavy metals can inhibit enzyme production
that helps our body convert thyroid T4 hormones into active T3. Since
our thyroid only makes 10 percent of the T3 our body needs, that conversion is essential for our endocrine and metabolic systems to function
properly.

In theory, at least farmed fish eliminate mercury. But like industrialized meat, there's the issue of transparency. In Asia, especially, the reports of shrimp and tilapia being raised in industrial waste water and fed
a diet of pig feces makes a little extra stress hormone like ractopamine
seem calming by comparison.

So where did this leave me for the remaining few weeks of anti-
inflammatory eating?

Just as I didn't want to give up all carbs, I knew that going the extreme route of becoming a vegetarian wasn't an option, especially now that said carbs were limited to whole grains. Buying better-quality meat at all times was expensive and not always possible when at restaurants. And in a country where a YouTube video of someone eating a 50-ounce all-bacon hamburger gets more views than the State of the Union, it was often difficult to rein in the portions.

In weighing the lesser of two inflammatory evils—processed grains versus industrialized animals—I decided to just try to make sure I was always avoiding one or the other and to pay more attention to how I felt after each type of meal.

The Sweet Spot

Food can be medicine and it can be poison. Our body knows what's best for us and it can also be our undoing. Our cravings are primal, and yet they're manipulated in a myriad of modern ways.

I already knew all this before I started my wellness project. What I didn't know was how to make those judgment calls: when to heed my body and when to ignore it; how to follow the siren call of the food angel on my shoulder and in my stomach, and when to throw the devil a candy cane–shaped bone. A big part of finding the middle ground between health and hedonism was learning when I could afford to cede control and be flexible and when my body dictated that I couldn't. In the case of gluten, it took a little tabbouleh to make me understand that even in the highest-stakes situation for my hedonism— gaining the acceptance of Charlie's family—I couldn't compromise my health.

For those with celiac disease, the daily choices around gluten are a no-brainer. If speaking up is a matter of life or death, you don't question the when or how, you just do it. My subtler symptoms—like the bloated belly and fatigue I experienced after dinner at Charlie's father's apartment—had given me the leeway to ignore them more frequently than I should have. It wasn't for lack of tuning in to my body. Rather, it was my love of food and fear of being a problem child that often inspired me to muscle through.

Finally understanding the downstream effects of my autoimmune disease made me realize that staying away from gluten was a nonnegotiable. Even if I only had one slipup every few months, the lasting effects meant that my system was at war year-round. However, I also recognized that stressing about the inflammation caused might be just as corrosive as the gluten itself.

Health food shame is a very specific kind of gut guilt. To indulge in something you crave or feel obligated to eat, knowing it will cause your body harm in more ways than just the numbers on a scale, can leave you feeling like a particularly bad person.

After the tabbouleh incident, I berated myself for not speaking up—maybe even more so than my immune system did. It made me wonder if perhaps forgiveness is the most anti-inflammatory ingredient we could feed ourselves.

There are so many food evils we face on a daily basis—many of which I grappled with during my clean-eating month. I found that the easiest way to sort through them, without losing my love of eating, was to instead focus on the good.

I'd always tried to eat a vegetable with every meal. But during my experiment, I saw how the proportions on my plate changed to put the colors of the rainbow front and center. If I made quinoa "fried rice," I was sure to add a pile of rainbow chard to offset the taupe specks in my wok.

The lack of hard carb-free rules allowed me to embrace my cravings in smarter ways—with plates of baked antioxidant-rich sweet potato fries, in addition to handfuls of spinach.

Dairy was less of a pain point. It was more of a garnish or seasoning—not an essential part of the blue plate special that I was raised on. I didn't have to grapple with not feeling full without cheese, and I knew the types and quantities I could get away with going forward without feeling sick. A little plain Greek yogurt or kefir, a few pats of grass-fed butter, and the occasional summer ice cream cone was a sweet spot I'd already found.

When I had a meal that included grains, I tried to make it vegetarian. And if I opted for meat, especially if it was questionable quality, at least I knew if I made the rest of my plate Paleo, with plenty of vegetables, that I'd be doing my blood sugar a favor. In doing so, I inadvertently tackled another digestive directive on my wellness to-do list: food combining. By separating starches and proteins, I was simplifying the number of tasks my gut had to perform to break down my meal—and I noticed feeling fewer urges to take a nap under the table afterward.

Eating different foods is important. They just don't have to be eaten all at the same time.

By the end of the monthlong trial period, my overall energy started to improve. It wasn't as dramatic a difference as the vice detox. But I was willing to take a longer route around Health Mountain if it meant eating in a way that felt intentional, not obsessive. When I saw Heidi again, she said my pulse no longer felt like there was a rave happening in my bloodstream.

There were a few times, in addition to my taqueria night, when I found myself embracing a YOLO clause—you only live once, girl!—or

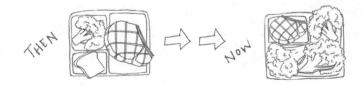

drifting from perfection in favor of not being the fussy one among friends. Straying didn't necessarily make me feel good either, but I tried to be kind to myself when my diet floundered in the face of life. Gluten was my only hard line, and for the rest, going forward I could embrace a little bit of wiggle room. A piece of millet toast or bowl of quinoa pasta wasn't going to derail my body in the same way as a plate of flour-dusted French fries. Like an isolated night of drinking, I could recover from a few spicy tuna rolls or a trio of mystery meat tacos. And I now had a clearer picture of what I needed to eat the following day to reset.

When I ate out, regardless of what I ordered, the combination of alcohol, hidden sugar, bigger portions, and richer food weighed on my body. Already having some skillet skills was a huge advantage that made eating cleaner much less of a struggle. But I knew that I still had a lot of room for improvement in turning cooking for myself into a consistent habit. If I could take back more control over my meals at home, then I could find more flexibility out in the world. And part of that was learning to cook better food, for less.

Here are some other tactics that will help you have a healthier relationship with food and eat better in the process.

1. *Keep a food journal for two weeks.* Food journals can be an amazing source of accountability and "aha" moments. As I discovered during this challenge, we often have selective memories about the junk we eat. A journal holds a mirror up to your actions, and the threads of food sensitivity may be so obvious that you can see them just by staring at the page. Otherwise, there are plenty of professionals—nutritionists, doctors—who can help you analyze the results. Writing down what you eat can also be a gateway to obsession, so use the journal as a short-term tool.

2. *Go on an elimination diet.* One of the most common sources of inflammation is a hidden food sensitivity. Try cutting out gluten, dairy, corn, soy, and sugar for two weeks (protocols like Whole30 and Autoimmune Paleo include even more foods). Reintroduce each item one at a time—leaving two days in between—with a large helping of the food in question. The heavy dose will force your body to give a clear reaction. This diet may seem extremely restrictive in the short term, but it will save you a lot of trial and error down the line. If you find you tolerate dairy, you can find your sweet spot going forward without depriving yourself forever just because someone told you it's "bad."

3. *Make your meals 50 percent vegetables.* You probably didn't need me to tell you that. But it's the common takeaway from pretty much every health protocol. Ideally, this will mean less

room on your plate for simple carbs and animal protein. But even if you're choosing to indulge, have a simple green salad as a starter before your steak frites arrives. Colorful antioxidant-rich veggies alkalize your stomach in advance of more inflammatory choices.

4. *If eating carbs, choose complex carbs.* Gluten-free doesn't necessarily mean healthy, especially when it comes to highly processed packaged foods. Pasta made from brown rice flour is healthier than bleached white flour, yes, but eating a bowl of whole brown rice is far better. In general, whole foods—meaning literally whole foods cut into pieces and not pulverized by an industrial grinder— keep your blood sugar down and your gut bacteria happy, while simple carbs, though easy to digest, cause more long-term inflammation.

5. *Go meat-free on Mondays or One Part Plant.* By reducing your animal intake, you forgo harmful hormones, heavy metals, and other inflammatory properties in the process. Try for one plant-based day a week, then eventually, one plant-based meal a day. This small change can also have a big environmental impact. You save more water by eating one less pound of beef a week than by not showering for six months!

6. *Don't substitute animal protein with soy products.* This is particularly important for my Hashi Posse, as soy can suppress thyroid function. A couple of splashes of tamari is one thing, but a big bowl of edamame or stir-fried tofu can throw your hormones out of balance. Opt for almond or coconut milk in your smoothies, and beans or legumes in your stir-fry if you're really worried about getting enough protein. If you do go for tofu, adding an iodine-rich ingredient like seaweed can offset some of the effects.

7. *Buy high-quality animal products.* The beauty of eating less meat means you can afford to invest in better meat. Buy organic, grass-fed, and free-range whenever possible. Avoid processed products like sausage, salami, and deli meats, which have been classified by the World Health Organization as carcinogens. For seafood, the best species for omega-3s, low mercury, and environmental impact are mollusks (clams, mussels, oysters, scallops) and smaller oily fish (sardines and anchovies). Wild salmon is also worth the premium. Limit your intake of tuna and swordfish to once a week. And if you do eat these high-mercury fish, add cilantro! It's a chelating agent that will help your body better remove the toxin.

8. *Don't let the food be the enemy of the company.* This tip comes by way of Megan Kimble's memoir, *Unprocessed: My City-Dwelling Year of Reclaiming Real Food.* She discovered (like me) how hard it is to have a restrictive diet outside the four walls of your home. Learn the things that you can be flexible around (a corn tortilla) and the things you can't (a bowl of tabbouleh). Because believe it or not, there will be times when you forget to bring your own beet chips to a Mexican restaurant. Always let hosts know your needs far in advance and offer to contribute to the meal. Look up restaurant menus prior to eating out, and even call ahead to get your questions answered in private to prevent a panic order.

VEGAN QUINOA "FRIED RICE" WITH RAINBOW CHARD

Serves 4

This healthier version of your favorite Sunday night Chinese take-out order is a great way to enjoy whole grains without letting them dominate your plate. The quinoa is balanced out with an even larger helping of vibrant rainbow chard, brightened up with fresh lime juice and a dash of Asian hot sauce, and "fried" using high-heat, hormone-friendly coconut oil.

....

1 cup uncooked quinoa, rinsed

$^1/_2$ teaspoon sea salt

2 tablespoons gluten-free tamari

2 tablespoons freshly squeezed lime juice

$^1/_2$ teaspoon sriracha, sambal olek, or your favorite Asian hot sauce

1 bunch of rainbow or red chard

2 tablespoons unrefined extra-virgin coconut oil

2 large shallots, thinly sliced

4 garlic cloves, minced

1 tablespoon minced fresh ginger

Hemp or sesame seeds, for garnish

1. In a medium lidded saucepan, combine the quinoa, $^1/_2$ teaspoon salt, and 2 cups of water and bring to a boil over high heat. Cover, reduce the heat to low, and simmer for 15 minutes, or until the liquid is absorbed and the quinoa is soft and pearly. Uncover, remove from the heat, and fluff with a fork.

2. Meanwhile, in a small mixing bowl, combine the tamari, lime juice, and hot sauce.

3. Separate the thick chard stems from the leaves and finely chop. Stack the leaves on top of one another and roll up like a cigar. Thinly slice into ½-inch ribbons.

4. Heat the coconut oil in a large wok or skillet over high heat. Sauté the shallots and chard stems until they begin to soften and caramelize, about 5 minutes. Add the garlic and ginger; cook for 1 minute more, until fragrant. Add the chard leaves and stir-fry until wilted and soft, another 3 minutes. Season lightly with salt. Fold in the quinoa and stir-fry until everything is evenly distributed and the quinoa is beginning to toast, about 2 minutes. Stir in the tamari, lime juice, and hot sauce mixture and remove from the heat.

5. Transfer to a serving bowl and garnish with hemp or sesame seeds for more fiber.

HEALTHY HEDONIST TIPS

Fried rice (even if you're not using actual rice) is best with stale, day-old grains. The drier they are, the more flavor they'll soak up without getting mushy. You can prepare the quinoa the night before, or make this recipe with 3 cups of leftover cooked grains, beginning at step 2. If you're the type of person who orders too much takeout, this would also be a great way to use up that half-eaten carton of brown rice and make you feel better about the previous day's food choices.

MARKET SWAPS

Any leafy green would work in this recipe: arugula, kale, collards, beet greens. If you're an omnivore or a v-egg-an, feel free to add 2 beaten eggs, like in a traditional fried rice recipe, at the end of step 4. Push the grains to the sides of the wok to form a well. Add the eggs to the center and scramble until set. Stir everything together, being careful not to overly break apart the omelet.

BAKED SWEET POTATO FRIES WITH COCONUT OIL—SRIRACHA AIOLI

Serves 2 to 4

As Michael Pollan writes in Food Rules: An Eater's Manual, *"There's nothing wrong with special occasion foods, so long as every day is not a special occasion." Deep frying is one of the most labor-intensive kitchen tasks, and before restaurants got involved, that used to deter us from indulging in fries more often than we should. Alas, this dish remains my biggest guilty pleasure, and since most restaurants don't use a dedicated gluten-free fryer, I've learned to make the next best thing in the oven at home.*

....

2 medium sweet potatoes (about 1 pound), scrubbed

2 tablespoons olive oil or melted coconut oil

2 teaspoons potato, corn, or arrowroot starch

$1/2$ teaspoon sea salt

$1/2$ teaspoon smoked paprika

For the aioli:

2 large egg yolks

1 teaspoon Dijon mustard

1 tablespoon freshly squeezed lime juice

1 teaspoon sriracha

1 small garlic clove, minced

$1/4$ cup olive oil

$1/4$ cup coconut oil, melted and cooled slightly

$1/2$ teaspoon sea salt

1. Position the racks in the upper and lower thirds of the oven and preheat oven to 425°F. Line two rimmed baking sheets with parchment paper.

2. Using a sharp chef's knife, cut the top and bottom off the sweet potatoes and stand them on one of the flat sides. Cut each into thin planks, ¼ inch thick, and then into matchsticks. Add the potatoes to a large mixing bowl and toss with the olive oil. Sprinkle with the starch, salt, and paprika; toss until well coated.

3. Divide the fries among the prepared baking sheets and arrange in an even layer, making sure there's space between each fry. Bake for 20 minutes, swapping the baking sheets from top to bottom halfway through, until nicely browned (but not blackened at the tips). Remove from the oven and toss the potatoes to redistribute. Return to the oven for about 5 minutes, until crispy. Allow to cool for a few minutes on the pan before transferring to a serving platter or 8-inch parchment paper cone.

4. While the fries are baking, make the aioli: In a small mixing bowl or bowl of a food processor, whisk or pulse the egg yolks, mustard, lime juice, sriracha, and garlic until smooth. Working slowly, add 1 teaspoon of the olive oil and whisk or pulse until incorporated. Repeat with 3 additional teaspoons. Once the oil is emulsifying easily, slowly drizzle in the remaining olive oil, followed by the coconut oil, whisking or pulsing throughout until thick. Season with the salt.

5. Serve the hot fries alongside the coconut oil–sriracha aioli for dipping.

HEALTHY HEDONIST TIPS

Sriracha is one of the few packaged condiments that I buy. I love the balance of flavors, and even though sugar is a line item, the amount is negligible. And as the residents who protested against their neighborhood sriracha factory's spicy fumes can attest, it's not really something you want to be making in your backyard or kitchen. Mayonnaise, on the other hand, is very easy to whip up from scratch, as I do in this recipe using hormone-healthy coconut oil. If you want to substitute store-bought, simply combine ⅓ cup with the lime juice, sriracha, and garlic.

MARKET SWAPS

To meet my anti-inflammatory color guide, I use sweet potatoes instead of regular spuds, but the technique works well for both. Since they become sticky once soft and roasted, sweet potatoes benefit from having a little starch added to help them crisp. If you're staying away from corn, try arrowroot or potato starch instead. You can omit entirely if you're using regular potatoes.

SKILLET SKILLS

BECOMING MY OWN PERSONAL CHEF

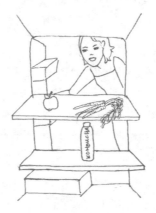

On preparing cleaner meals, without being a slave to the stove.

ate one Tuesday night toward the end of my anti-inflammatory eating month, I arrived home after teaching a cooking class with the type of relief and exhaustion that comes from hours of being on your feet, talking with your hands, and monitoring every movement to make sure no one amputated an index finger.

The windows hadn't been cracked all day, and being in a stuffy, confined space made me more aware of the faint smell of food drifting in from the hallway. *My neighbor must have made stir-fry tonight*, I thought. Until I realized the waft of charred onions was coming from my own hair.

I'd spent the whole subway ride home thinking about the kale salad I had been paid to demonstrate, not consume. And now I was standing at the edge of the low-blood-sugar abyss, one step away from a meltdown.

I opened my fridge to take in the scant offerings, a result of working more in other people's kitchens rather than my own. Eggs, half a box of limp arugula, the remains of a two-pound bag of now-hairy carrots, and a Tupperware container of plain cooked white beans stared back at me.

I had more than enough to throw together a meal and I knew exactly what I'd make with this mystery box challenge. But it was late, I was tired, and my hunger pushed all productive cooking thoughts from my mind. So I did what I always did in these ill-prepared off-hour situations.

I got Thai food.

A few celebrity chefs like Seamus Mullen and Marco Canora, who've had their own reckonings with autoimmune disease, have spoken about how people who spend all day taking care of others are often the worst at taking care of themselves. I had noticed this trend in my own behavior as I began cooking more professionally. There's nothing like lugging twenty pounds of someone else's groceries twenty New York City blocks to make your biceps want to pick up the phone instead of a frying pan to get dinner on the table.

The fact that every day of my workweek as a self-employed food babe was a different beast was one of the reasons why so many of my self-care practices had slipped since leaving the corporate world. There were no more predictable six a.m. trips to the gym and six p.m. visits to Whole Foods. Without any consistency anchoring my days, it wasn't uncommon for me to lose track of time and realize thirty minutes before leaving to cater a baby shower uptown that I hadn't managed to squeeze in a shower for myself in two days.

As much as I wish my life were an endless Instagram feed of morning acai bowls, bespoke shaved carrots with pea microgreens, and relaxed afternoons reading *Bon Appétit* on my vintage chaise, I am not that person. If I were, I probably wouldn't need a year of wellness experiments to help me feel like less of a mess. Instead, my sink contains a perpetual stack of crusty prep bowls, making the idea of dirtying more cookware to fix myself a last-minute dinner seem exhausting. And as a result, prior to anti-inflammatory eating month, my body's cells probably consisted of 20 percent pad Thai.

My latest challenge had helped me reconnect to the idea of eating intuitively and, in the process, pulled back the curtain on how some of my favorite comfort food was actually making me feel. My latest delivery order had included a sensible and restrained combo of veggie green curry and brown rice instead of syrupy noodles and not-grass-fed beef, but the unrestrained way in which I inhaled them left me in a fugue state on the couch for hours.

It was clear that cutting ties with my containers of Thai delicacies was a necessary next step.

In many ways, cooking is a habit-forming activity, just like going to the gym: you have to be willing to set aside some time in the kitchen if you want to eat better. I had the skills, the fully loaded pantry (complete with southwestern lamb seasoning and jalapeño chutney), and the random scraps of vegetables dying a slow death in my crisper drawer. Yet, on most nights, instead of cobbling together a last-minute stir-fry at the stove, the convenience of my Seamless app was often too strong to ignore.

In the past, I'd found that it was easiest for me to commit to cooking in one long session over the weekend—when I actually had the leisure time to enjoy it. I decided to run with this batch-cooking strategy for my next wellness sprint: every Saturday or Sunday I'd spend a few hours preparing meals for the week ahead. It might take some planning, but I knew nothing could curb my take-out habits better than always having homemade food at my fingertips. And I hoped that the ritual of reheating it would be stronger than my current ritual of ordering from an app, or eating beet chips with hummus on the couch and calling it dinner.

Alone in the Kitchen with a Piece of Salmon

I was lucky to have grown up in a household where food was routinely cooked at home, and kitchen skills inadvertently trickled down to me.

My mom was the original gangster of crunchy health food. She knew full well that when an industrial factory is producing your food, it tends to mix in a lot of junk (like vital wheat gluten) that normal people would never add to their dinners, even in the most egregious Paula Deen recipe. Growing up, she shopped almost exclusively at a place called Mrs. Greens, which had shelves of organic fruit leather that was just a touch too leathery, bulk bins of various carob-covered nuts, freezers full of Rice Dream ice cream, and checkout counters stocked with blond-dreaded employees who smelled vaguely of cedar chips. The snack food brands available at this store were not those advertised during commercial breaks of *Salute Your Shorts*. So naturally, I spent most of my childhood rebelling against my mom's moratorium on the cottonseed oil in generic packaged foods by going over to friends' houses and having a Fruit by the Foot free-for-all.

My attitude change began the summer of high school I spent working the front desk at a fashion magazine, living at home while my parents were away for the summer. To ensure that I had enough of my allowance saved for the important things—like lip gloss, Michael Stars T-shirts, and weed—I turned to the random grains and petite-diced tomatoes in my mother's well-stocked pantry.

I remember very vividly standing in the kitchen with the cordless phone in one hand, spatula in the other, asking her how long I was supposed to cook a piece of salmon for, and was it bad that the fillet was frozen solid when I put it in the pan? These early experiments yielded unfortunate results, many of which required the assistance of a few condiments to make them palatable. But by the end of the summer, after I had blown through all of the frozen fish and was down to her last can of chickpeas, I had gained a special appreciation for the unglamorous-yet-satisfying art of throwing together a meal from cans, jars, and freezer bags.

I realized that, in recent years, I had lost some of this resourcefulness.

Like my bathroom cabinets, I had successfully hoarded the entire bulk-bin section of Whole Foods, yet I rarely started there when planning recipes, whose endgame was to be topped with superfluous garnishes and photographed on a scrap of burlap on my floor.

It wasn't the weekend yet, but so I wouldn't have to resort to takeout again, I decided to get a jump start on this challenge by making a few meals using only what I had on hand, just like that summer in high school.

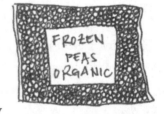

There were already a few moments during my project when I saw that, with every healthy baby step, I was slowly realizing the universal horror of becoming my mother. But when I opened my freezer, it was clear that the metamorphosis had begun long before I started scanning labels for added sugar and cottonseed oil.

Inside were bags on bags of frozen vegetables, Tupperware containers stored with Tetris-like precision, and a few individually portioned wild salmon fillets, impulse-purchased during a sale months prior. Like the frozen blueberries I'd discovered during the vice detox, much of the contents of this petrified graveyard had been long forgotten.

I took out some peas, trying to remember which bag I'd previously used as an ice pack, and left the salmon to defrost in a warm water bath.

To use up the wayward vegetables, which were looking too sad to be eaten on their own, I put a pot on the stove to make a batch of desperation soup. Hoarding clearly runs in the family, and this is my uncle Denny's favorite weekly strategy for emptying the fridge: throw everything together, add some seasonings, and simmer until it becomes a luscious melting pot of united flavors. I'm pretty sure this is also how the Tuscans created their first minestrone soup. I dumped in the white beans and a can of tomatoes and called it that.

IN A STUDY published by *The American Journal of Clinical Nutrition*, researchers found that meals prepared at home were followed by "more intense, positive emotions and less worry" than those eaten outside the house. Besides the calorie argument, there's something to be said for what cooking does for your happiness.

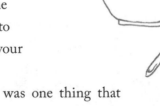

For me, that feeling of comfort was one thing that made the habit stick.

Back in high school, being on my own gave me the freedom to indulge in things I would have never eaten in front of another human— things like a bowl of defrosted peas with half a stick of butter (and a scandalous splash of white wine from the liquor cabinet). And it also allowed me to embrace the learning curve in a safe space, knowing that if the brown rice somehow turned out to be both undercooked and burnt at the same time, as it often did, no one would be around to judge.

As I stood alone in the kitchen, I realized that it had been a while since I cooked a meal at home that didn't have anything to do with brand work, blog posts, Charlie, or friends. It was nice not to have anyone around to impress—or even the Internet—and I was reminded how satisfying it was to make something simple like a bowl of frozen peas with butter and white wine (for old times' sake) and a fillet of fish (now that I actually know how to make one well), as a special gift to myself.

Money Doesn't Grow on Organic Apple Trees

Becoming your own private chef for a month is admittedly a lot easier when you happen to already be a private chef.

I'd had a lot of practice cooking many make-ahead meals in a single afternoon. I'd basically been doing this challenge once a week for the last three years—just not for myself. When cooking for clients, though, I was used to having a carte blanche to fill my canvas totes with however much grass-fed filet mignon I wanted. But when it was my credit card at the checkout counter, I had a harder time wrapping my mind (and wallet) around how much higher-quality ingredients actually cost.

Like investing in sustainably raised animals, many of the medical voices in the autoimmune community, along with my extremist endocrinologist, said that buying organic produce was necessary if I wanted to fully heal.

"We now have lots of evidence that pesticides are not just toxic; they are particularly likely to trigger an autoimmune condition," writes Amy Myers, MD, in *The Autoimmune Solution*. One study comparing the death certificates of three hundred thousand farmers found that those working with pesticide-treated crops were more likely to die of an autoimmune condition.

Instead of being rigid about seeking out labels that said "organic" on them, I knew I'd be better off just shopping exclusively from the farmer's market.

For most people, myself included, going to the grocery store can be a stressful experience—they're designed to accost your senses with new impulse items at every turn. It's hard enough to know what to buy without the added task of trying to find food that's actually as healthy as its packaging claims. Having gone through the circus of greenwashing when shopping for my natural beauty products, I knew the lure all too well.

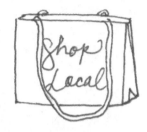

Over the years, I'd learned how to turn my blinders on and stick to the store's perimeters (where the produce, meat, and seafood counters usually are), but at the farmer's market, I could avoid pesticides, hormones, and antibiotics without having to overthink it. Even if a stand isn't certified organic, most small farmers who aren't pushing out supermarket quantities tend to use more sustainable growing practices. And unlike conventional vegetables—which travel an average of fifteen hundred miles to get to your kitchen table—buying locally shortens the time between harvest and consumption, meaning more nutrient bang for your buck.

Still, that didn't mean the farmer's market didn't have the potential to become a money pit. Between the huckleberry jams and artisanal duck prosciutto, I'd often left with a canvas tote full of expensive impulse buys that were hardly the building blocks of an actual meal.

To keep myself in check, I decided to limit myself to forty dollars. I would put two twenties in my pocket and leave my purse at home. This budget didn't seem unrealistic if I was trying to make four or five dishes, enough for a week's worth of lunches and a few solo dinners.

My catering work had taught me how important it is to begin any shopping trip with a plan in place. So I took another inventory of my pantry and drafted a rough menu of building blocks I could mix and match: one meaty stew, a lentil-based main, a simple roasted vegetable, and a dark leafy salad. While I would have ordinarily listed out every specific ingredient, I wasn't quite sure what produce the market would have that Saturday.

With budget and availability providing extra wildcards, I would have to face this first batch-cooking challenge at the farmer's market flying by the seat of my yoga pants.

Farm to Table

The Union Square Greenmarket in New York City is usually a whole foods circus. Warm weekend afternoons require a situation-room-level plan of attack to get past the throngs of ambling tourists and fedora-clad locals, preciously sifting through bins of fiddlehead ferns.

On this freezing spring morning, however, the regular market-goers seemed to have decided to hole up at home with their Chemex carafes and seven-grain loaves from markets past. The offerings were reduced from the usual length of three city blocks to just a small corner. And I could tell that even the shivering farmworker replenishing the fingerling potato crate was secretly dreaming of moving to Palm Springs.

I grabbed a bunch of deep garnet beets, a couple of sweet potatoes, some loose knobby carrots, and a head of red cabbage roughly the size of my own dome. I hesitated when I saw the meager remains in the kale bin. But as someone grabbed one of the last three bunches, a wave of farmer's market FOMO hit me and I pounced.

With my first twenty-dollar bill nearly spent, I headed to the meat and seafood counters. I knew that this was where my budget would start feeling pinched. I wanted to make sure I had enough left over to get a dozen eggs, their vibrant amber yolks definitely worth the premium price. When bought fresh at the farmer's market, eggs can last for weeks, making them a great fridge staple. A little leftover quinoa "fried rice" might seem like a meager lunch offering. But put an egg on top? Now you've got bulk and novelty and yolk porn. And those yolks, in addition to being an Instagram gold mine, are also the best source of choline, an essential nutrient for women during childbearing years.

As I browsed the freezer case full of grass-fed beef and heritage pork chops, I was again reminded that forty dollars wouldn't get me very far if my idea of dinner was an 8-ounce steak in the middle of my plate, though the ostrich filets were surprisingly affordable. Ordinarily, I might have chatted with the butcher and tried to find some cheaper odd cuts, but my fingers were beginning to lose feeling. I grabbed a more familiar quart container of ground chuck and went home to thaw out over my stove.

A Spoonful of Butter Helps the Vegetables Go Down

Back home, I immediately started rinsing, peeling, and trimming vegetables.

Prepping is where everyday races against the clock are won or lost in the kitchen. Adopting a more efficient workflow by assembly-lining one ingredient at a time shaves off many minutes, and means fewer distractions once fire is involved. The chef-y term for this is "mise en place," which is just a fancy French way of saying "get all your ducks in a row before you start actually cooking."

As I de-stemmed the greens, I was pleasantly surprised by how many fresh ingredients I had managed to buy. I dressed the kale and roasted the carrots. I cooked the beets, topped them with toasted almonds, and used their greens to add some leafy goodness to a batch of quinoa. I stretched the 12 ounces of grass-fed ground beef with a can of black beans from my pantry and added some cubed sweet potatoes to create a big pot of comforting chili. Finally, I split that hulking head of cabbage and turned half into a spicy slaw and braised the rest with French lentils, red wine, and butter—a humble peasant dish that my Jewish relatives would probably refer to as "shtetl food."

FAT HAS GOTTEN a bad rap over the years as a macronutrient more widely associated with cankles than a balanced diet. But the tide is starting to turn.

"All forms of sugar (with small and relatively insignificant differences) have the same negative effects on the body," writes Mark Hyman, MD, in *Eat Fat, Get Thin: Why the Fat We Eat Is the Key to Sustained Weight Loss and Vibrant Health*. "[But] not all fats are to be vilified, and eating liberal amounts of the right ones will not make you fat."

Today, even the American Heart Association has eased their cholesterol restrictions, urging people to cut back on added sugars and embrace good fats instead. Charlie forwarded me an article that announced these new guidelines as proof that his heart would be just fine with a few extra slices of bacon. I tried to explain that the fats they meant were those found in olive oil, avocados, nuts, seeds, fish, and whole eggs—a very different story than the trans fats in processed foods or saturated fat in certain meats. Still, I often found myself using his indulgent preferences to my advantage.

Butter may still be controversial in the medical community, even if some sides of the wellness world laud it as a superfood. But in terms of effectiveness, I'd argue that a little goes a long way in making healthier items like cabbage and lentils something a pickier eater might actually want. It gives less popular nutritional all-stars the assists they need to score. Which, as I discovered back in the day with my peas, is what healthy hedonism is all about.

Other than an innate preference for sweet over bitter, most of our food likes and dislikes are learned. And there are two main strategies that have proven successful at getting kids on board with broccoli: repeat exposure and flavor masking, a Mary Poppins–esque technique that harnesses the power of tastes that you already like (sugar, butter) with things that you might not enjoy yet (peas, cabbage).

At an event around the time of these cooking experiments, I happened to meet a prominent bariatric surgeon who was one of the more outspoken haters of saturated fat. To weigh the cost and benefit, I asked him: if it takes a pat of butter to get someone to eat their vegetables, is it better to skip the butter or the greens?

"Eat the vegetables," he grumbled.

I had planned on eating most of my preprepared meals by myself since Charlie was working late for most of the week. But come Friday night, when the chili had long since run out, I was surprised to see him happily inhaling my shtetl food, which had just a big enough spoonful of butter to make the lentils go down more easily.

Good and Cheap

Having prototyped my clean make-ahead meal plan on two consecutive weekends at the Union Square Greenmarket, which has an impressive, if relatively expensive, selection, I was worried that my new routine might just be the pipe dream of a jaded New Yorker. Would I have been able to cook the equivalent spread—a satisfying array of five different veggie-centric dishes—if I lived in an area with fewer fresh options? And would I have been able to do it for forty dollars without the crutch of my overloaded pantry?

Luckily, I was about to find out what it would be like to put the forty-dollar batch-cooking challenge to the test outside my organic golden triangle of Whole Foods, Trader Joe's, and Fairway.

During the slog of holiday catering season when I was getting close to no creative work done, I had applied on a whim to a writers' colony in the mountains of Tennessee. I thought it would be a good way to escape the frenetic energy of the city, but in the midst of said energy, I had nearly forgotten about it when the acceptance email landed in my inbox. I would be heading down south at the end of the month.

Though I wasn't overly optimistic about finding a farmer's market nearby, with no Thai takeout for twenty miles, it seemed like the perfect opportunity to see what healthy cooking on forty dollars a week was like in the heartland of America.

DESPITE ALL THE *Top Chef* marathons and Cronut fetishes, Americans spend less of their income on food than any other place in the world. Most of our policies are designed to produce calories as cheaply as possible. That alone, however, isn't responsible for our lack of spending proportional to other consumer goods. People in wealthy countries like France and Japan spend about double what we do on food—14 percent of all consumer expenditures each, compared to our 6.7 percent. Why do we invest so little of our paycheck in something so essential?

Before I left for the south, I sat down with Leanne Brown to get her thoughts on our country's collective food budget.

Leanne became an expert on what it actually takes to cook healthful meals on SNAP food stamp benefits, which she talks about openly, honestly, and practically in her best-selling cookbook *Good and Cheap: Eat Well on $4/Day*. As part of the food studies program at NYU, she compared ingredient availability and prices at various grocery stores in New York City with data from around the country and then developed recipes to help people with tight budgets eat better.

"People should probably spend more," Leanne said, taking a sip from a single-drip coffee that probably cost more than the daily cooking budget of her project. "But at school, this conversation just seemed like such a middle-class concern. I felt like there were these fifty million people whose voices just weren't being heard. And it really bothered me."

Friends in the program were blown away by how good Leanne's food was—just as good as, if not better than, the things they were making with much more flexible means. It made her realize that kitchen skill, not budget, is really the key to eating well. So she decided to write a cookbook for her final project, and after putting up a campaign to raise money for print copies—with a TOMS Shoes–esque buy-one-give-one model for families in need—her cookbook became the most successful one ever funded on Kickstarter.

I wanted Leanne to tell me if my assumptions were right that packaged food wasn't always cheaper than its fresh, from-scratch counterpart before I had those assumptions beaten out of me by the Manwich cans in aisle three.

"Unless you take into account the cost of your time, there's no way prepared foods are cheaper," Leanne said. "There are some things that take longer that may never be worth bothering with. But pancake mix? You're one step away from making something from scratch, and what comes out of the package sucks a hundred times more."

For people who have so little money to work with (a budget of four dollars a day), cooking from scratch can make your grocery bill a lot more affordable. But there's still the issue of the time required to prepare meals. After talking to families on SNAP, Leanne realized how much less of it they had to play around with in the kitchen, compared to the luxurious hours I spent honing my skills in my mother's organic playpen.

"In many ways, I think people who have very strict dietary restrictions face a similar type of fear as those with monetary limits," she said. "If you mess up something with your diet, you might be too sick to go to work the next day. For people on SNAP, there are similar consequences if you take a misstep with your groceries: you might not be able to put dinner on the table tomorrow. It can take a lot of the joy out of preparing food."

Her shopping tips, which focus on buying cheap bulk pantry items like grains and beans, and opting for frozen vegetables if fresh aren't available, try to make the tough choices around dinnertime a little more bearable and give people some freedom from the budget side of the "what's for dinner?" question.

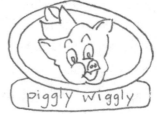

A lot of her advice was not unlike the strategies I'd already used during my make-ahead meals challenge at the farmer's market. Even at the regular grocery store, buying in-season ingredients helps you save money.

"You'll pay a lot more if you want to make a peach coffee cake in February," she added.

This Little Piggy Went to Market

I kept some of Leanne's tactics in mind as I pulled up to the Piggly Wiggly on my first morning in Tennessee. It was the main game in town, and as I began browsing the small corner devoted to produce, I couldn't help feeling a little bratty and homesick.

Assuming the organic options would be limited, I had tried to brainstorm recipes around items that fell under the Clean Fifteen. Of the samples tested by the US Department of Agriculture, these were the fruits and vegetables (avocado, mango, asparagus, and onions, for example) that were least likely to contain pesticide residues, while the Dirty Dozen consisted of the biggest offenders (berries, apples, tomatoes, cucumbers, and peppers). For instance, the average potato had more pesticides by weight than any other vegetable, while sweet potatoes were on the safer side.

I was never going to be perfect on the organic front, but I could do my best to avoid the most pesticide-heavy produce. I added some sweet potatoes to my cart, along with broccoli, onions, garlic, ginger, and a box of organic spinach, and continued on to the meat section.

As my eyes grazed the rows of shrink-wrapped chicken tinged the same yellow as the logo slapped across the package (thanks to their all-corn diet), I began to worry that I'd have to rely on vegetarian dishes for the entirety of my stay if I wanted to avoid antibiotics and hormones. Eventually, I stumbled upon the one organic option: a roll of 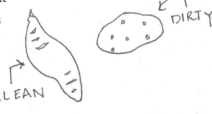 frozen ground turkey in a dark corner of the freezer section, next to gluten-free chicken nuggets and soy veggie burgers. At ten dollars, it was exorbitant by the Pig standards. But even with the produce and a couple of pantry items—chickpeas, canned tomatoes, brown rice—I only went over budget by a few dollars.

The writer's kitchen was stocked with olive oil and a haphazard array of spices that past residents had left behind, but aside from an impressive selection of bourbon, there were no quick-fix pantry items that could be consumed as is. For two weeks, I would have to rely completely on my from-scratch skills, three meals a day.

The spices came in handy for adding variety. I used a little smoked paprika to turn the can of chickpeas, wilted spinach, and tomatoes into a rich Spanish stew. The cumin and cayenne allowed me to re-create that comforting go-to chili with ground turkey, which I ladled over twice-baked sweet potatoes later in the week. And the brown rice, sautéed with ginger and broccoli, became a bed for countless fried eggs for breakfast, lunch, and dinner.

The market selection may have been less plentiful and the veggies less bespoke than what I was used to, but at the end of my time in Tennessee, I didn't end up eating much differently than I might have at home. In fact, without any factory-farmed chicken in my take-out orders, my two weeks of cooking from the Piggly Wiggly were arguably healthier than any weeks leading up to my cooking challenge. And they were a welcome reminder of what good home cooking can do to balance out the occasional tumbler of bourbon.

The Sweet Spot

My health seemed to be coasting on a higher plane since switching up my eating habits.

During anti-inflammatory month I tried to keep the hedonism in my meals through beet chips and brown rice—by adding a handful of good, so I could still enjoy some of the bad. Only, in doing mental math around my diet, I sometimes forgot to find the joy in my food.

Focusing on problem solving in the kitchen—with time and budget as my main contingencies—made me feel much more in sync with what I was eating. And not just because I was aware of the ingredients and where they came from but because cooking forced me to slow down and rediscover my passion and purpose in the process.

Food is so much more than just fuel. It's ritual and culture, something to be savored and celebrated. It's a way of spending time with a family member from afar, reliving memories, or stepping into the shoes of your sixteen-year-old self without having to put on a pair of Steve Maddens.

When you cook, there's more that feeds you than just what ends up on your plate: the smell of sweating onions; the small, scalding samples from a wooden spoon along the way. Carving out time for cooking filled me up in more ways than one. And because of the effort involved, I took pride in the accomplishment. Even if I was just reheating leftovers, I found that I was eating in a more controlled way. It was a very different experience from pouncing on a plastic take-out container and inhaling. Sometimes I used food as a means of procrastination, which could turn my lunch into a bottomless bowl. I felt a lot less like a manatee after meals during my batch-cooking experiment.

It also made me less wasteful. I was much less likely to chuck the fruits of my prior labor than a half-eaten container of congealed rice noodles that it took five minutes to source. Once I began investing in higher-quality perishable ingredients at the farmer's market, I had an even bigger financial incentive not to let them die a slow death in my crisper drawer. The beauty of planning ahead and cooking all those dishes in one afternoon meant I didn't have the scraps that make so many beginner home cooks feel wasteful when they first get started in the kitchen. My budget forced me to buy fewer veggies and use them start to finish.

When I prepped my produce on Saturday afternoon, I used a bowl to collect any compostable scraps—fennel fronds, carrot peelings, garlic skins, herb stems—as I sliced and diced. Every part of the vegetable contains flavor, even if it's not necessarily the most pleasant part to munch on. At the end of my cooking session, I added those scraps to a ziplock bag and stored them in my freezer.

Determined to no longer use this drawer as a veggie burial ground, at the end of the month I dumped my frozen bits and pieces into a giant pot, along with some dried herbs from my spice rack, and made a month's worth of "recycled" veggie stock, creating something for free—for future desperation soups—that I might have otherwise bought.

THE FOOD GIFTS you give yourself, it turns out, don't have to be such a production. Batch cooking was an important reminder not to let perfection be the enemy of good. And that there's something to be said for

embracing a few modern conveniences—
like the microwave—that make our time
in the kitchen less of a chore.

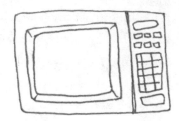

Toward the end of the week, when my
farmer's market bounty was down to its
last few bites, the hedonist in me still
craved some corners to cut in order to make cooking more sustainable.
Which is part of the reason (in addition to cravings) why I returned to
eating some gluten-free processed grains (bread and pasta) when in a
pinch.

I still loved whipping up an indulgent dinner for Charlie, or submit-
ting to my creative whims with a batch of Brussels sprout latkes that took
hours to shred and fry. But this challenge helped me get a grip on my
everyday habits.

Shopping and eating on a budget meant learning to embrace and reuse odds and ends. Preparing multiple dishes in a single cooking session
meant learning to love some of the humble one-pot recipes that make up
so many ethnic cuisines. And crafting meals from leftovers on a day-to-day
basis made me smarter about adding last-minute accents, like an oozing
coconut oil fried egg.

The beauty of local produce is that you don't need to gild the lily to
make it delicious. Roasted vegetables from a nearby field with olive oil
and sea salt is one of the simplest and most gratifying dishes on earth.
And that's the kind of easy cooking ritual anyone can get behind.

Healthy Hedonist Cooking Tips

You don't need to go to culinary school to become your own personal chef—I didn't! Here are some tricks of the trade, though, that will help you build better cooking habits and be smarter about the time and money you do spend at the stove.

1. *Set aside a weekend afternoon to cook for the week ahead.* Use the first hour to do the majority of your prep work—clean and chop produce and get your ingredients organized. Aim to use the next two hours for cooking and a third for cleanup. If you have a buddy or partner, you will be able to make your meals for the week in even less time!

2. *Always make a menu, budget, and shopping list.* Designing your menu around existing items in your pantry and fridge—just as you would a seasonal ingredient at the farmer's market—will help save you money and cut down on waste. If you're cooking everything at once, choose dishes that can be made with a variety of techniques—that is, a mix of roasting, stewing, and raw, instead of four dishes that require the stovetop. An ideal breakdown is a couple of one-pot meals (stews or soups), a produce-centric bowl of grains or legumes, and one or two easy vegetable sides. (For more tips and menus, see Appendix C on page 350.)

3. *Use your freezer as an economical extension of your pantry.* Can't make it to the store every week? Stock up on frozen vegetables! Your freezer also allows you to take advantage of fresh seasonal items on sale. If there's a special on wild sockeye salmon, bring home some fillets and freeze them individually for future

use. There are some canned items that I could never swear off (tomatoes, for one), but frozen is generally healthier as you avoid the toxic BPA (bisphenol A) lining that's in most cans (another known endocrine disruptor). Trader Joe's and Eden Organics are two great brands that use BPA-free cans.

4. *Diversify your animal intake.* Unfortunately, a cow is not made up of all filet mignon, and the sea is not 70 percent salmon. Ask your butcher or fishmonger to recommend some other (cheaper) options. Since they're used to going home with the stuff no one else wants, they're a wealth of cooking knowledge. Better yet: buy the whole animal. Labor always gets added to the price tag. Bone-in chicken thighs will be cheaper than boneless. And bringing home the whole chicken is by far the cheapest way to go.

5. *Buy in bulk.* Just like the labor in deboning chicken breasts, you end up paying a premium for packaging. Pulling straight from the bulk bins allows you to buy just as much or as little as you need and pay by weight—this is where I source all my whole grains, nuts, seeds, and dried fruit. Store them at home in mason jars or other glass storage containers. Bulk buying also applies to packaged goods. You may not be making puttanesca sauce tonight, but if you see a sale for capers, anchovies, or canned tomatoes, it pays in the long term to stock up when these shelf-stable items are at their cheapest.

6. *Use your spice rack.* This is one of the best places you can put your money in terms of creating flavorful meals out of humble ingredients. Suddenly, one cup of lentils can become five different dishes. Spices also have amazing medicinal powers. You can slowly build your collection up over time, but many will lose their punch and efficacy after a year or two.

7. *Make "peasant" food.* The Romans in particular were incredibly frugal: think stale bread in meatballs, Parmesan rinds in soup. A lot of Asian cuisines use meat as more of a garnish (ahem, pad Thai) instead of as a centerpiece, which is both healthier and cheaper. If you're making many dishes at once, it helps to stick to one ethnic cuisine for your menu so you can mix and match throughout the week. Once you have all the condiments, making takeout at home becomes that much easier.

8. *Invest in good-quality fats.* Coconut oil is the healthiest fat for frying because it has a high burning temperature. Heart-healthy olive oil is great for low-heat cooking or as a topping for salads and roasted vegetables. Grass-fed butter is a luxury, but, as I mentioned, you can't beat it for flavor.

9. *Avoid nonstick cookware.* If you're going to spend money on organic vegetables and grass-fed meat, don't cook it on something just as harmful as pesticides! Teflon pans contain PFOA (perfluorooctanoic acid) in their nonstick coating that becomes toxic when very hot (go figure). If you're using these pans, cook dishes like scrambled eggs or omelets, which require only a low flame, and avoid metal spatulas that will tear the coating. Better yet, replace them with inexpensive, long-lasting cast iron. It will be completely nonstick if cared for properly.

10. *Ignore expiration dates.* Americans throw away 165 billion dollars' worth of food every year. One reason: hysteria around grocery items that have exceeded their expiration dates. Don't rely solely on these numbers, which are arbitrarily set by the brands themselves, which benefit from you buying more food. Instead, look for signs that something has gone off. If it smells fine and has no

visible mold, you're usually good to go. And if that mold is on cheese, cut around it and nibble away.

11. *Use your veggie scraps.* Recycled veggie stock is a great way to reuse onion skins, herb stems, and the like. Some other ideas for often-tossed parts: asparagus stalk pesto (page 308), pickled chard stems, and candied lemon peel. A little garlic and a quick sauté can save even the saddest bruised salad greens. Or just make Desperation Minestrone Soup (page 131).

12. *Brown bag it.* If you're the type of person who goes out often and feels home cooking gets in the way of your social life, commit to bringing lunch to work. As Mark Bittman acknowledged in his protocol VB6, your daytime meals are when you have the most control and willpower to make good choices. Start by batch cooking just two dishes for the week. Pack them individually and put a note on your door so you remember to take them in the morning.

13. *Get a farm share.* If you're committed to weekly batch cooking, a CSA (Community Supported Agriculture) is one of the most affordable ways to get large quantities of local produce without having the hassle of going to the farmer's market. Many will deliver directly to your door. The less often you go to grocery stores with a million impulse options, the less you're likely to stray from your healthy food choices and budget. There are also mail-order services, like Thrive Market, that offer healthy, responsibly sourced pantry items at conventional prices thanks to a membership model.

DESPERATION MINESTRONE SOUP

Serves 4

What do you do when you have overflowing bowls of veggies that are about to go south? Throw them in a pot. The end result will most likely be comforting for your countertops and your spirit. Rustic minestrone soup is a great strategic base for your desperate times of produce abundance. I'm pretty sure Italian peasants invented it as a haven for whatever scraps were left over at the end of the week. I've given very loose instructions so that you can account for whatever is in your crisper drawer on any given Sunday.

....

1 tablespoon olive oil, plus more to drizzle

1 small yellow onion, diced

2 cups finely chopped pantry vegetables (carrots, fennel, leeks, potatoes, cauliflower, cabbage, winter squash, etc.)

2 large garlic cloves, minced

One 15-ounce can diced or crushed tomatoes

8 cups vegetable or chicken stock

1 teaspoon salt

$1/4$ teaspoon red pepper flakes

One 15-ounce can cannellini beans, drained and rinsed

1 cup finely chopped green vegetables (zucchini, green beans, peas, leafy greens, broccoli, etc.)

$1/2$ cup gluten-free elbows, orzo, or orecchiette (optional)

$1/2$ cup fresh herbs (basil, chives, parsley, tarragon, or a combination), coarsely chopped or torn

Shaved Parmesan or pecorino, for serving (optional)

1. Heat the olive oil in a large Dutch oven or stockpot. Sauté the onion and pantry vegetables over medium-high heat until soft, 5 to 7 minutes. Stir in the garlic and cook until fragrant, another minute. Pour in the tomatoes and simmer until the liquid is reduced and the tomato chunks have softened, about 5 minutes. Add the stock, salt, and red pepper flakes to the pot. Turn the heat to high and bring to a boil.

2. Stir in the beans, green vegetables, and pasta (if using), then reduce the heat to medium-low. Simmer for 10 minutes, or until the pasta is cooked through. Remove from the heat, stir in the herbs, and taste for seasoning. Garnish with a drizzle of olive oil and shaved Parmesan or pecorino for a salty bite.

HEALTHY HEDONIST TIPS

When I'm in the mood for a little more protein, I start by browning ½ pound of organic chicken or turkey sausage at the beginning of this recipe. Processed deli meat and precooked sausage are often loaded with harmful preservatives, but a little sustainably produced, fresh hot or sweet Italian sausage from the butcher counter is a great option. You can also easily make your own sausage by combining ground chicken or turkey with fennel seeds, red pepper flakes, and dried Italian herbs.

MARKET SWAPS

This recipe is meant to be an edible way to compost all your wayward produce. Pantry vegetables are the sturdy ones that last a while in the crisper drawer of your fridge. The green veggies cook quickly, which means you should add them toward the end of the soup process. Another great addition from the garbage bowl: a Parmesan or pecorino rind to add a rich, cheesy flavor to the broth. Next time you finish a wedge, save the rind in your freezer until it's soup time.

SKILLET RED-WINE BRAISED CABBAGE AND LENTILS

Serves 4

Breaking into my mother's liquor cabinet—if only to cook some peas—gave me a real thrill as a rebellious teenager. Little did I know that my scandalous splash of white wine cooked off as it simmered. The same goes for these braised lentils, so the dish doesn't fall too far into hedonism territory. The only naughty aspect comes from a pat of grass-fed butter, which offsets the tangy wine and cabbage. But I could eat these lentils all day long even without it. Don't be intimidated by the braising time: the recipe is fairly hands-off and a good one to have in your batch-cooking repertoire, as you can prepare other dishes while it simmers.

....

2 tablespoons olive oil

1 large red onion, sliced

$1/2$ small (1 pound) head of red cabbage, thinly sliced ($2^1/_2$ cups)

2 garlic cloves, minced

1 cup dried French green lentils, rinsed

2 sprigs fresh thyme or $1/2$ teaspoon dried

$1^1/_2$ teaspoons sea salt, plus more if needed

1 tablespoon Dijon mustard

2 cups dry red wine

1 tablespoon organic unsalted butter (preferably grass-fed), plus more
   if needed

1. In a large heavy-bottomed skillet or Dutch oven, heat the olive oil over medium-high heat. Add the onion and cabbage; cook, stirring occasionally, until the onions are translucent, about 10 minutes.

2. Add the garlic, lentils, thyme, and salt. Cook for 2 minutes more, until fragrant. Stir in the mustard and spread the lentil-cabbage mixture in an even layer. Pour in the wine and 2 cups water (enough to submerge the lentils). Bring to a simmer and cook over medium-low heat, stirring with a wooden spoon every 10 minutes or so, until the lentils are tender and the liquid is mostly absorbed, 45 minutes to 1 hour.

3. Remove the skillet from the heat and stir in the butter. Taste the lentils for seasoning and add more salt (or butter!) as necessary. Serve warm with a side salad.

HEALTHY HEDONIST TIPS

Pantry hoarding goes for the liquor cabinet as well. This recipe is a great way to use up week-old wine or that rogue bottle brought to your house-warming party. The recipe calls for 2 cups, which means there's still a little nip left for you if you open a new bottle.

MARKET SWAPS

Diced beets and their greens would be a great swap for the cabbage (or in addition to it), since you don't have to worry about their color bleeding everywhere (the braising liquid is already red). To make this a meatless main, add a fried or poached egg on top. And if your picky eaters require some meat in the mix, brown 1 pound of chicken thighs before step 1. Set it aside and about 10 minutes before the lentils are done cooking, nestle the meat in the cabbage mixture.

WATER WORKS

FILLING MY WELL

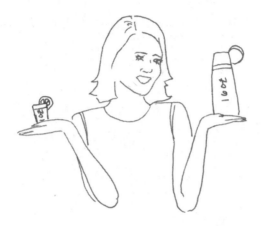

On creating a hydration habit with better, purer water and more of it.

D*rink more water* is not the sexiest of wellness manifestos. For many, it falls under the category of common sense. Yet so many of the experts I talked to when designing my curriculum—and even my own naturopath endocrinologist—cited chronic dehydration as one of the biggest barriers to good health.

You would also think that it's one of the easiest and cheapest issues to fix. But there are many things that get in the way of hydrating *right*. And the first is that most people don't reach for water in the first place.

Since the first month of my project I had gotten better at scanning food labels for brown rice syrup, fruit juice concentrates, molasses, and maltodextrin—among the fifty other names for sugar. But I was less discerning when it came to beverages, especially with those thought to have added nutrients.

As soft drinks have become public enemy number one, giants like Coke and Pepsi have started pushing smaller "healthy" brands. Take coconut water, for example. Since the category started expanding a decade ago, it's become a four-hundred-million-dollar business with claims that drinking it can cure kidney stones, improve skin, fight infections, and super-hydrate you post-workout.

While these drinks are a step in the right direction away from sodas, they aren't necessarily better than—or even as good as—plain old H_2O. Coconut water may have added minerals that help your cells take in water, but it also has only slightly fewer calories per fluid ounce than Gatorade. A recent study (ironically funded by Vita Coco) also found that neither coconut water nor sports drinks were better than plain water at hydrating post-workout. So why was I spending my money on raw, organic coconut water and pretending I was doing it for my body instead of my sweet tooth?

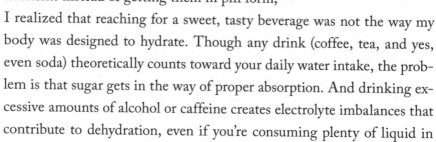

Just as I knew that I should eat my nutrients instead of getting them in pill form, I realized that reaching for a sweet, tasty beverage was not the way my body was designed to hydrate. Though any drink (coffee, tea, and yes, even soda) theoretically counts toward your daily water intake, the problem is that sugar gets in the way of proper absorption. And drinking excessive amounts of alcohol or caffeine creates electrolyte imbalances that contribute to dehydration, even if you're consuming plenty of liquid in the process.

Taking a closer look at my food budget during both of my clean-eating challenges, I realized how often I impulse-bought hibiscus green tea or chia strawberry lemonade while waiting in the mile-long checkout line at Whole Foods. These drinks had become a loophole in my low-sugar anti-inflammatory program. And now that I was on the way to getting my diet under control, I wanted to make sure my drinking habits weren't shooting my eating habits in the foot.

I needed a challenge that would get me back in the habit of making regular, flavorless H_2O my healthy drink of choice. And the best way to do that—and balance my budget in the process—was to stop spending money on other drinks in the first place. For a month, I would try to drink my daily water quota and ban buying all other beverages, with the exception of tea, wine, and whiskey (on the rocks).

Quenching Your Thirst

Without any distractions for my taste buds, the next step was to figure out exactly how much water I should be drinking.

I had a hunch that the eight-glass-a-day adage was an oversimplification and I quickly learned that the more accurate rule of thumb is to drink half your body weight in ounces daily—even more if you live in a dry place or exercise a lot. Many doctors recommend that you also pay attention to some secondary cues: drinking until your pee is consistently the mellowest of yellows or until you no longer feel thirsty.

The latter, though, was something I'd always wondered about.

In college, I remembered reading a magazine article about how our bodies often mistake thirst for hunger. It was most likely in a piece on weight loss, and I probably only held on to the information as a way to talk myself into drinking a can of Diet Coke instead of inhaling multiple packets of Raisinets during bouts of late-night studying at the library. Nevertheless, the tidbit stuck with me.

Hunger is something I'd gotten pretty good at recognizing. If I missed the growls from my midsection, I could usually rely on the irrational rage that set in, which subsequently prompted me to think about when my next period was due, and then consider the last time I'd eaten. Charlie had also gotten adept at reading the warning signs, so much so that he sometimes put a breakfast bar in my hand before I'd had the chance to do either of those things.

Thirst, though, was much more abstract. I had never experienced a hangry equivalent extreme enough to cause my significant other to pour a beverage down my throat out of fear.

It's not necessarily that our survivalist instincts have weakened over time. Rather, in modern life, the differences between liquid and solid nourishment have gotten so blurred that the lines between thirst and hunger often get crossed in 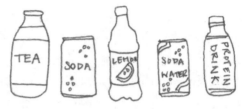 the lateral hypothalamic area of the brain. Today, our beverages involve added calories (soda, juice), while our actual food is often in liquid form (soup, smoothies). And then there's the tendency to reach for a no-calorie soda as a way to ward off cravings for real food.

The perfect storm of hunger-thirst confusion is Diet Coke. Caffeine stimulates the brain, even if it's exhausted, causing it to overuse energy reserves. With normal soda, some of that energy is supplied in the form of sugar. With artificial aspartame—which is two hundred times sweeter than sucrose—the hunger craving gets doubled: the sweet taste signals to the body that more energy is on the way, but the replenishment never comes. It's a huge rush of promise, followed by no actual nourishment.

Learning this made me wonder how many times in my tweendom I had staved off midday hunger or late-night study munchies with a diet soda, and wound up back at the vending machine an hour later inhaling Smartfood popcorn at fifty kernels per minute.

Liquid Courage

The most commonly recognized symptom of dehydration is a headache—usually, the sledgehammer variety you experience after a night of too many margaritas. I was reminded of this uniquely miserable sensation on more than one occasion after my vice detox as my body tried to remind me once again that I was no longer twenty-two. But my crowning moment of hangover hell came right before I started my water experiments.

Now that I was at the five-month mark of my project, it was interesting to see where my habits aligned on the healthy hedonism spectrum. With sugar and caffeine, I had been more successful at finding moderation. My taste buds had dulled since the wedding night macaron binge once some added sugar was brought back into my life, but I was still more sensitive to sweets than I had been. I could tell whether a product had added sugar in it without even looking at the package. The one time I ate pad Thai since my clean-eating experiment, I couldn't taste anything beyond the tangy sauce that clung to each rice noodle.

This new sensitivity also extended to synthetic smells. Having rid my routine of so many artificial fragrances, I was acutely aware whenever any infringed on my airspace. When I went to get a haircut, I found myself wanting to borrow a surgical mask from the colorist painting dye onto the roots of the blonde next to me. It was hard to sit near friends who wore too much perfume at dinner or watch as my host lit a scented candle in the middle of her tablescape, the smell of artificial lemon verbena eclipsing the intoxicating rosemary beef stew in the middle of the table.

Thanks to the farmer's market challenge—which I was trying to continue—my eating habits at home were much improved. The order history on my Seamless app revealed that I was now only averaging one take-out order a week, which felt like a small victory. And being better about cooking made me less stressed about the additives that could be lurking in my food when I wasn't fully in control of my meals.

Weekend brunch was still my time to indulge in eggs, bacon, and bloodies. And when there were expertly roasted hipster coffee beans around, I added that indulgence to the list. If I sipped slowly and limited myself to one small cup, I didn't usually feel jitters as I had when gulping down coffee alongside a blueberry breakfast cupcake.

The area where I struggled the most with moderation was with alcohol. I had slipped back into old bad habits now that the weather was warmer and people were emerging from their chunky-sweater hibernation. With my social calendar packed, it was back to the casual and unnecessary Monday night glass of wine with friends. Back to letting Charlie open a bottle for our weekday date night meals at home. And back to feeling like shit after we exhibited no self-control and drank the whole thing. I couldn't tell if it was an issue of tolerance or just added awareness, but even one glass of wine seemed to propel me into a fog that lasted twenty-four hours.

It was rare that I partied beyond the scope of wine-filled dinners. The problem was that when I did, I didn't know my limits. Because in a matter of months they had changed.

ON A FRIDAY NIGHT in early May, Charlie and I found ourselves pressed shoulder to shoulder in a large swarm of teenagers wearing neon American Apparel crop tops. It was a well-known concert venue that both of us had frequented in the past. But never before had we felt so, well, old.

We were there to support one of Charlie's friends who, after years of DJ-ing college bars and cancer benefits, was now riding the momentum of a top ten single. It had been a long week of work, and we were both already experiencing the onset of claustrophobia and sensory overload.

"We should do shots," Charlie screamed in my ear, barely audible over the opening act. The rest of the group agreed, sensing that the night would need to be chased with a good dose of tequila.

It had been a while since I'd had a wild, unrestrained night of hard liquor. And with every sip of well alcohol, my body seemed more at ease with the beat, the bouncing NYU students, and the glow-in-the-dark beach balls being punted at my head. By the time the main act assumed their throne in 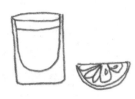 the middle of the stage, I was no longer wishing I had brought earplugs or worn sneakers. I was barely even aware I had ears or legs.

When it was over, we stumbled the twenty blocks back to Charlie's apartment, bumming a menthol cigarette from another concertgoer on the way, and regressing even further into the disorderly behavior we'd outgrown ten years prior. The next thing I remember was the bathroom door hitting me on the side of the head with a dull wallop.

"Get up," I heard Charlie whisper from somewhere on the other side of it. I was sitting on the toilet, where I must have passed out, folded over my legs like a retired marionette. "You need to move," he repeated more urgently. "I'm going to be sick."

I used the sink to pull myself upright, and the second I had ceded my position, Charlie dropped to his knees and began retching. The sound prompted my mouth to turn on like a warm faucet, and without further warning, I was bent over the sink, its shallow basin doing little to contain a barrage of tequila and partially digested pasta.

"I think it was the cigarette," Charlie groaned around noon when we finally awoke to the piercing afternoon light pouring in from his bedroom window.

"Right," I said. "Definitely just that."

I spent the next forty-eight hours in a hangover apocalypse. No attempts at hydration would undo the damage.

Your Body's Many Cries for Water

As I started reading up on the long-term effects of dehydration (and believe me, there's no drier topic on the planet), it didn't take me long to stumble upon the work of Dr. F. Batmanghelidj. Despite the fact that his book *Your Body's Many Cries for Water* was harder  to get through than *Ulysses*, it's sold millions of copies worldwide.

In it, Batmanghelidj claims that our failing thirst mechanism, coupled with the wide availability of "hedonic" beverages such as soda, have caused a dehydration epidemic of massive proportions.

Many of us think that serious dehydration only happens after an extreme activity like running a marathon or drinking too much tequila (and then regurgitating it). But Batmanghelidj argues that gradual everyday water loss can cause an equal amount of ongoing insidious damage to your system, even if we can't recognize these symptoms as thirst.

He discovered the healing powers of water in a rather nontraditional setting: an Iranian jail. While serving as a political prisoner, Batmanghelidj treated three thousand of his fellow inmates suffering from stress-induced ulcers with the only "medicine" he had—water.

When I read this, I wondered how many of the health ailments Charlie consistently complained about could be caused by dehydration. But upon further investigation, there didn't appear to be a whole lot of official research the good doctor did once he had escaped Iran and started proselytizing the "Water Cure" stateside. The medical community has since written off his claims as nonsense, including a lengthy peer review on QuackWatch.org.

I wanted to do the same. But on the other hand, I didn't think scaring people into drinking more water was the worst thing in the world. Doing so might not have prevented my grandparents' Alzheimer's disease any more than not eating carbs would have. Water is not a cure-all. But as more recent research has revealed, not getting enough can very well cause long-term harm in the form of kidney stones, cholesterol problems, liver issues, and joint or muscle damage. One study (albeit with a small sample size) even found that dehydrated drivers made twice as many errors during a two-hour commute—a statistic not terribly far off from driving drunk.

Could some of my body's issues be a result of lasting, insidious dehydration? A week of trying to drink half my weight in ounces illustrated how often I probably failed to do so.

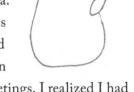

During the first week of my water challenge, I used a big pitcher to measure out my daily quota. On the days I was home, I refilled my water glass constantly as a healthy form of procrastination and blew through my first 30 ounces by noon. But when I was cooking for clients or running around to meetings, I realized I had gone entire afternoons without so much as a sip of anything.

As I struggled with two heavy bags of groceries, I wondered: could my sporadic cranial throbbing simply be my body crying out for water? Recently, several studies have shown that regular headache sufferers' symptoms lessoned when they drank water. Perhaps when you take an aspirin for that bad back or headache, the water you swallow with it helps just as much as the pill.

According to a Harvard study, half of American children are dehydrated. The average adult drinks just 20 ounces of water a day—not even close to the recommendation. (The average adult male weighs 196 pounds, meaning he should be drinking 98 ounces per day.) If our cells are slowly losing water, is it that far-fetched to think there might be other ailments as a result?

Dehydration should be easy to treat. But how can you fix a problem you don't know you have?

Survival Instincts

The first time I experienced serious non-hangover-related dehydration was in my midtwenties when I found myself, against all better judgment, on a reality cooking show. Even though I come from a family of serious *Survivor* enthusiasts, it's a fun fact that still makes me squirm.

The casting notice came at the end of a real doozy of a year. I had just painfully parted ways with my best friend and writing partner, leaving a giant void in my personal and professional life. My other long-term relationship was hanging on by a thread, but given all the shake-ups in my corner, neither of us had the guts to break out the mercy scissors and cut the other loose. Like many reality contestants before me, you could say that I was adrift enough to feel like I had nothing to lose. And had I not lost my North Star in multiple areas of my life, I probably wouldn't have ended up in the Colorado wilderness with cameras following me as I foraged for prickly pear and cattails.

The show was a mash-up of several other successful concepts and involved two teams of chefs traveling across the country, trading cooking skills for food, transportation, and shelter. I was excited to have the opportunity to prove to my parents that when the cameras were off, their favorite contestants were out back loading up on the network's best catering services. Unfortunately, though, reality TV life was realer than I'd expected, and I spent the majority of my seven-week tenure borderline starving.

During the Colorado challenge, we were given shelter in the form of tents on the side of a mountain, but we had to forage, shoot, or catch all of our food. By the end of my first day, after an unsuccessful afternoon of hunting prairie dogs in the summer heat (because it was the only thing in season), I hadn't put anything except water in my body for twelve hours. I was starting to feel dizzy and, despite not being there to "make friends," I worried about seeming weak in front of my tattooed teammates. God forbid they think my nausea was caused by having to field dress a rodent.

Nature won that round, though, and soon I was hunched over the side of a cliff watering whatever cattails and prickly pear lay below with stomach bile.

The producers sensed this plot twist was more pathetic than dramatic, and I was quickly carted off to a cabin a few miles away. For the next twenty-four hours, I slept on a couch under a hypothermia blanket, being intermittently woken for a dose of Gatorade and bananas by our mountain guide, Rooster.

It didn't occur to me at the time that I was seriously dehydrated. For one thing, vomiting and diarrhea, two extreme forms of expelling liquid, seemed like counterintuitive ways for my body to tell me I needed water. Plus, I had been consuming plenty of it in place of actual meals.

What I learned the hard way in Colorado, with no Bear Grylls to guide me (just a guy named Rooster), is that if you're bingeing on water alone, you end up flushing out a lot of your sodium and other essential minerals. And that can be just as bad as having too little water in the first place.

Hydration is a complicated, delicate dance. And even back in real life, I turned out to be just as uncoordinated at it as the tango.

With a Grain of Salt

The year following the show was when my health really started to decline. The initial improvement I felt once I stopped eating gluten quickly unraveled along with a good chunk of my spirit. It was nice to temporarily escape to the nonreality of reality TV—rifles, prairie dogs, and all. But once I came home to the emptiness of my actual reality, an overwhelming loneliness set in.

I shed a good amount of water weight via my tear ducts that fall. I had finally cut the cord with the boyfriend, and the heaviness of losing two best friends in one year began to slowly stifle any desire I had to leave the apartment. So I dipped into my usual breakup routine of '90s rom-coms and bland foods whose tastes wouldn't remind me of a million sad-face emojis when I ate them again months later.

Whether or not it was fueled by depression, my body seemed to have a harder and harder time summoning the effort to get out of bed in the morning. I also noticed that increasingly throughout the day, my hands and feet would start to tingle with numbness, my fingers so pale, purple, and cold to the touch, you'd think I was back in the Colorado wilderness, this time digging for tubers in the snow.

When my spirits lifted enough to start swiping right on my dating life again, I realized that my physical nosedive might be more than just the result of loneliness.

It had been five years since my Hashimoto's thyroiditis diagnosis, and five years that I continued to stubbornly go without hormone replacement medication. Eventually, I found an endocrinologist to address some of the issues that were probably not caused by sadness.

. . .

DR. A WAS exactly what you'd expect from a Greek naturopath: sun-kissed bushy hair, tanned skin, missing-in-action lab coat, and a Shih Tzu to keep you company while she reviewed your new-patient intake forms.

After going through my blood work and rattling off items 1 through 20 of her recommended dietary protocol, she reviewed a few other prongs of my medical history. "You have a lot of back pain too, yes?" Dr. A asked rhetorically. "Well, look at these numbers. You're chronically dehydrated! Do you drink water?"

"Actually, yes," I said, thinking that this was one of the few things I was doing right.

"Good, good. But you're not absorbing it properly. We need to work on your adrenals."

Dr. A explained that these little glands, also in the endocrine chain of command, are in charge of regulating the body's stress response through adrenaline and cortisol, our chief fight-or-flight hormones. When the thyroid is out of commission—as mine had been for over five years—the adrenals have to work extra hard to generate energy for the body. While my thyroid ran on fumes, I had unknowingly been barreling full speed ahead 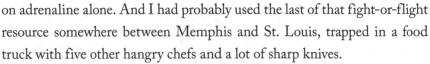 on adrenaline alone. And I had probably used the last of that fight-or-flight resource somewhere between Memphis and St. Louis, trapped in a food truck with five other hangry chefs and a lot of sharp knives.

Adrenal fatigue for overworked New Yorkers, especially women, might be as prevalent as the common cold. But a side effect that few people recognize is dehydration.

Since the adrenals sit just above your kidneys, their other main function is to control your water levels. The more stress you have, the more hormones and salt they send out to circulate in the body. When your stress levels fall, all that sodium needs to be evacuated. Just think of a nervous Shih Tzu puppy that has to pee all the time. That's the stressed-out you, constantly flushing fluids, along with sodium, down the toilet.

As I learned in Dr. A's office, people with adrenal fatigue can drink their full daily water quota and still be dehydrated. And since I was one of them, she sent me home with a bottle of liquid electrolytes that would replace some of the sodium and minerals my fatigued adrenals were discarding. My bag also contained three hundred dollars' worth of other pills, including B complex for my numb appendages and evening primrose oil to regulate my hormones (apparently it had done wonders for her dog's coat).

I had to buy three day-of-the-week pill cases just to keep up with my new regimen and switch to a larger purse to carry them all with me. Some supplements needed to be taken with meals, others on an empty stomach. As a result, I had to remember to take one capsule or another five times a day. It was a lot to wrap my head around. Especially a head already being addled by a special brand of Hashimoto's dementia.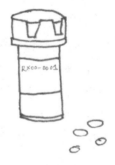

I took Dr. A's supplements as best I could for a few months. But most of the other lifestyle directives were lost on me.

You could say that starting my wellness project was a way of slowly making good on all of her advice. Only now, a year later, the healthy hedonist in me was learning to take it all with a grain of unprocessed sea salt, one piece at a time.

Soaking It All In

Now that I was finally whipping myself into water shape, I wanted to make sure that what I was drinking was actually feeding my cells.

My months of clean eating had helped break up my immune system's thyroid-shaped piñata party. And my latest round of blood work revealed that my antibodies were continuing to go down, even if certain vitamin levels still put me at risk for being a malnourished chef. Though much of the turmoil caused by Gloria the Healer's wheat germ supplements seemed to be behind me, I wondered if during that flare-up, when my thyroid was barely performing, my adrenals had begun to pick up too much of the slack again.

I was feeling good about how consistently I was finishing my daily water quota. But was it enough? Now on to applying some best practices for absorbing it properly:

1. Start the day with a big glass of water. The morning is the best time to hydrate since you've just gone eight hours without anything to drink. Adding fresh lemon juice, like I did during the vice detox, not only helps flush toxins, it aids in absorption by adding potassium and vitamin C to the mix.

2. Add a pinch of sea salt. Like fat, salt has gotten a bad rap in the age of processed foods, despite the fact that it's an essential nutrient. Salt is in the makeup of virtually all of our bodily fluids, which means we're constantly losing it in the form of sweat, urine, and tears. Perhaps I would have been better off nursing my heartbreak with a bowl of salty home-made sweet potato fries, instead of an entire pint of ice cream. Dr. A, along with many other functional medicine practitioners, recommend pink Himalayan or sea salt because it's less processed and thus retains important minerals that also aid in absorption and support electrolyte balance. I tried to add a pinch of it to my morning lemon water or smoothie.

3. *Sip slowly.* Think about your body's appetite for water in the same way as food. Just because you've had a big breakfast doesn't mean you're not going to be hungry again by dinnertime. Drinking a quart of water at the beginning of the day and then going dry for the rest is the same concept. What we don't need in a given moment gets flushed down the toilet, and our cells' thirst returns shortly thereafter, regardless of whether or not we can recognize it. I have a bit of a chugging problem, so I wanted to try to stop using my daily water intake as a conditioning exercise for future games of flip cup. I also wanted to think about having three good "water meals" a day: one 16-ounce glass before breakfast, lunch, and dinner.

4. *Drink when you're not eating.* It's good to have these "water meals" outside of your actual meals. To maximize retention, stop drinking thirty minutes before eating and wait an hour after you're done to drink more. This is a struggle, especially when you accidentally eat the ghost pepper in your Thai curry. But passing up water during a meal also helps with digestion. Water dilutes the natural enzymes in your saliva that help break down food and has a similar effect when it reaches your other digestive organs. Wine is metabolized differently, so the same rules don't apply. (Phew.)

5. *Focus on fiber.* While it's best not to drink while you eat, it's good to have some lingering fiber in your gut to help slow down absorption. This means that instead of washing straight through your system (like the contents of my CamelBak did in Colorado), your body has more time to take in all the water it needs. The best way to do this is to get some extra fiber in the morning. Think hemp seeds in your oatmeal, almond butter in your smoothie, or veggies in your scrambled eggs. It also means that a

chia strawberry lemonade is a better choice than a sugary beverage without any pulp or seeds.

I decided I would try to incorporate these concepts into my water routine for the rest of the month. But there was still one more big piece of advice that Dr. A stressed more than any other. And I definitely couldn't fully clean up my water act without addressing it.

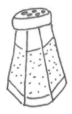

What's on Tap

Part of being a born and raised New Yorker, in addition to an affinity for bagels and sidewalk road rage, is being proud of our tap water. When out to eat, I always asked the waiter for "a bottle of the city's finest" in an attempt to be charming.

The more research I did during Project Hydration, though, the more I realized how outdated the regulations on public drinking water are. The list of banned chemicals hasn't been significantly updated since the 1980s, which means that under the Clean Water Act, rocket fuel additives and dry-cleaning solvent can still legally flow from our tap.

Especially after the crisis in Flint, Michigan, people often talk about the risk of lead and other heavy metals—a by-product of aging pipes and infrastructure—but I was equally disturbed to learn about the drugs. When we take prescription meds, as with excess salt and other toxins, what our body doesn't use gets flushed down the toilet in our urine. While this wastewater is treated before it makes its way to reservoirs, rivers, or lakes, and then again before it ends up back in the glasses of consumers, most treatment plants don't properly filter drug residue.

"Although research on pharmaceuticals in the water supply began almost a decade ago, no one seems to know which compounds need to be removed or how to remove them from the water safely," *The New Republic* reported in 2013. "And no one seems to know which government agency should step forward and take action."

In 2008, the Associated Press launched their own investigation and found drugs in the water of twenty-four major metropolitan areas, each having its own special mix of sex hormones, chemotherapy, and antibiotics. Southern California had particularly high levels of antianxiety medications, which might partially explain the laid-back vibe of its residents.

Of all of her views on my questionable wellness practices, Dr. A was perhaps the most flabbergasted when I told her I didn't filter my water and rarely, if ever, drank any H$_2$O that didn't come straight from the tap. The ingredient she was most concerned about was fluoride. Many people think it's a plus (fewer cavities!), but the substance added to 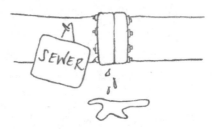 today's water system is a by-product of the aluminum industry and is very different from the naturally occurring calcium fluoride that was originally used. Sodium fluoride is one of the main ingredients in commercial pesticides and, along with chlorine, is particularly problematic for thyroid health. They both compete for iodine resources—an essential ingredient for the production of healthy thyroid hormones—and Dr. A told me I'd never be able to control my Hashimoto's while ingesting so much of them.

Unfortunately, though, I quickly learned that affordable, space-efficient pitcher filters like your standard Brita don't do an effective job at filtering some of the worst offenders. And because nothing ever comes cheap and easy in this toxic wonderland of ours, fluoride is by far the hardest one to remove. Reverse osmosis technology is the most reliable method, but it also takes hours to work its magic, wastes even more water than it produces, and strips what ends up in your glass of essential minerals. Plus, the top-rated options I came across would cost me several months of wellness slush fund money and much of my already limited counter space.

I settled on a solid carbon block model. For one hundred dollars, my new ten-stage water filter attached to my faucet and took care of the lead, chlorine, pharmaceuticals, and other big contaminants. It also only required a replacement filter once a year, which made it a more affordable and convenient option than a pitcher, whose cartridge I would have had to replace every two months.

I was happy to finally have a system at home. But, as with my natural beauty transition, once I knew all of the dirt on what was in our water, I had a hard time not feeling completely paranoid when I wasn't able to safely sip from my own filtered tap.

One night when I was out to dinner, the waiter asked his usual: "Tap, still or sparkling?" And in a moment of panic, I abandoned my old shtick in favor of something safe and packaged.

"Really?" my friend looked at me. "What's wrong with tap?"

I didn't have the heart to tell her. Suddenly, I questioned my decision not to go with New York's finest and hoped my glass was heavy on the Xanax.

Bottle Service

To make matters more confusing, it turned out that my dinnertime instincts were misguided. As I researched the healthiest water options when away from home, I discovered New York's finest might just be on par with Poland Spring—or even better.

Despite marketing claims, most bottled water is more likely to be sourced from a man-made well in Queens than a glacier in Alaska. In fact, it's estimated that half of all bottled water is actually just municipal tap water with a cuter outfit. And even water packaged from a more "natural" source isn't necessarily any cleaner. Unlike municipal suppliers, beverage companies aren't required to have their water tested by a certified laboratory. During a 2006 ad campaign, Fiji started talking smack about Cleveland's water supply, only to have the city fire back with evidence that the brand's water contained high levels of arsenic that was absent from their tap.

And then there's the small matter of BPA plastic bottles, which add even more endocrine-disrupting toxins to the liquids they house.

When I was in a bind, I could splurge on store-bought water that came in a glass bottle. Some brands now even sell water in a carton. While both of these materials are better for your body and the environment than plastic, the superior solution was to always try to travel prepared.

To feel better about the water I was drinking outside the house, I bought a cheap on-the-go filter for when I wasn't near my faucet. For ten dollars, I added a small Japanese activated charcoal stick to my portable bottle. These thin, porous logs look like something you pull out of a campfire, but they are surprisingly adept at absorbing impurities. Activated charcoal bonds with toxins on a molecular level, and it's the material used in most carbon block filtration systems. Even your trusty Brita uses granulated charcoal, hence the black bits at the bottom of your glass when the filter is on its last leg. Having the whole solid charcoal stick is a more eco-friendly alternative. They last for up to six months, fit nicely in a carry-on bag, and, once retired from their filtration duties, can find a second life absorbing the odors in your stinky fridge.

The Sweet Spot

I was pretty disheartened to learn that if I wasn't careful, I could be poisoning my body at the same time I was expending so much energy trying to purify it.

But, more so than with a lot of my other experiments, I felt like my water habits would easily stick. Now that I'd fortified my home against the hormones and other hazardous ingredients lurking in my tap, it was one less thing on this exhausting quest for wellness that I had to think about.

Once I started measuring out my requisite ounces (my body weight divided by 2), it was pretty easy to ensure I was meeting my quota. By the end of water month, I didn't even need to keep track anymore; I could remember if I'd skipped one of my water meals. But it always helped to have a glass in front of me as a visual reminder to refill.

The toughest part of my experiment was weaning myself off drinking water at meals. I missed it in the same way I still sometimes missed ending dinner with something sweet, now that I no longer stocked dark chocolate bars in the house. Without the palate cleanser, though, I noticed other flavors a lot more, specifically how salty and spicy my food was. Luckily, I was no longer eating much Thai takeout.

I still hadn't identified any of my body's cries for water that were as insistent as my hunger-induced meltdowns or hangover headaches, but I resolved to keep my system constantly afloat so that my insides didn't feel the need to use their outdoor voices to get my attention.

Once I had my new filter, I felt pretty silly for not having bought one sooner.

CHARCOAL STICKS $15

Just because you can't necessarily identify symptoms caused by the chemicals in tap water doesn't mean they don't exist. Especially with toxic metals like lead, exposure builds over time. It might have been too soon to tell if making this change had an impact on my energy, but I knew that overall, hydration month made my lips, hands, and face feel less chapped. And by getting my water meals through plain H_2O instead of sugary coconut water, my cravings evened out, proving in some ways that hanger could be tempered side by side with thirst.

After a month with my filter, I noticed that my sensitivity to smell now included water. At restaurants, I could tell if what was in my glass was tap before it even reached my lips. The top note of chlorine was as pronounced as the taste of cleaning fluid that was barely rinsed from the glass. Health reasons aside, the water from my filtered tap just tasted better.

I was curious, though, if other water omnivores would agree. So I conducted a not-so-scientific blind taste test to see if twenty of my friends could tell the difference among tap, bottled, and filtered water. Even though he had logged less time drinking water than anyone else I know, Charlie was convinced he would crush this exam. A few people got all the waters right and, annoyingly, he was one of them. But the more impressive result was that my filtered tap beat out the bottled water on taste. The data, I admit, was meager, but in my eyes it just strengthened the argument that bottled water is a waste of money.

Of course, there were always going to be times when I left the house without my reusable water bottle and had to buy some. Drinking impure water is better than drinking no water. Our livers are designed to be our own personal water filters and make sure toxins are eliminated properly. But none of our organs can properly function without any water at all. So when in doubt, I tried to relax and take a sip.

Healthy Hedonist Hydration Tips

Water is an essential ingredient in our body's health and also an amazing detoxifier. Here are some ways to fill your well more wisely.

1. *Treat all drinks other than water as you would alcohol.* Anything with calories from the beverage aisle should be considered a treat, like a glass of wine, and not something that your body actually needs. Soda especially should be a special-occasion indulgence, like a tequila shot. Coffee and tea are of less concern but shouldn't be considered part of your daily water quota.

2. *Put a water pitcher or bottle on your desk.* This not only helps you measure your daily intake, but it's also a powerful reminder to drink. If you don't want to count ounces at all, you can get a container that holds your exact daily quota.

3. *Infuse to add flavor.* As I learned from my partner in crime, not all of us are natural water enthusiasts. A little added flavor goes a long way. I like using fresh fruit, sliced cucumber, or herbal tea leaves. Making compound ice cubes is a great way to create that spa effect without breaking out a cutting board. I love the combination of lime juice and ginger (Ginger-Lime Ice Cubes, page 160)!

4. *Use charcoal sticks on the go.* Drinking clean water when you're traveling is a lot more difficult than making a concerted effort at home. A Japanese charcoal stick is a great, cheap, portable filter. The only catch is you need to let it do its thing for an hour to get the best results. They also need to be "refreshed" every few months,

which involves simply boiling them for ten minutes. You'll want to replace them completely every six months.

5. *Skip the plastic bottles.* Get a stainless steel or BPA-free reusable bottle to take with you on the go. When you consider that it actually takes three bottles' worth of water to manufacture a single plastic water bottle, it's even more clear that it's better to skip the endocrine-disrupting plastic that leaches into the water we drink, and then into the soil once we throw those bottles away. That said, if you're in a foreign country where there's a real question of potability, buy bottled water to be safe from pathogens.

6. *Buy a filter.* There's no need to immediately clear your countertops for the Ferrari of filters. It's best to start somewhere that's not going to put a drastic damper on your lifestyle or your wallet and upgrade from there. While pitcher options may seem the cheapest, make sure to calculate the annual cost. Soma, which makes beautiful sustainable carafes, is ninety dollars when you account for the six replacement filters you'll need for a year's use. This brand offers a subscription service for new cartridges so you never forget to replace them. For others, make sure to mark your calendar. Drinking water from an expired filter is more toxic than what comes out of your tap in the first place.

7. *Get one for your shower too.* You spend a lot of intimate time with water every day in the bathroom. Once I learned that skin can absorb up to eight glasses' worth of toxins during the average rinse, I immediately purchased a filter for my showerhead. It seemed silly to spend so much time and money obsessing over the water I drank if I was just going to be absorbing a comparable amount of chemicals through my skin.

8. *Use a fabric shower curtain.* Believe it or not, your shower curtain is one of the most toxic things in your home! The liner is usually made of PVC (polyvinyl chloride) plastic, which means you're hotboxing your bathroom with endocrine-disrupting phthalates every day. You have to wash a fabric curtain often if you don't want it to become tie-dyed with mildew, but I felt like this downside was worth what it did for my toxic load. You can always get a second cloth curtain to hang on the outside to help with aesthetics.

9. *Switch your shaker to sea salt.* Iodine is an important ingredient for good thyroid health, but too much of it can throw its function out of balance. It only takes a half teaspoon of iodized salt to meet your daily allotment, and if you're eating a balanced diet, chances are you're already getting this through fish, eggs, and vegetables. Keep unprocessed sea salt or pink Himalayan salt at home so you can control your iodine levels and gain plenty of other essential minerals.

10. *Make bone broth the new coconut water.* Bone broth is literally so hot right now. As animal bones simmer for hours, they release amino acids, collagen, and nutrients that help your body make the most of the liquid you put in it. It turns out that homemade chicken soup is just as good for your immune system as it is for the soul.

*For a full list of my favorite water products,
visit FeedMePhoebe.com/Shop.*

GINGER-LIME ICE CUBES

Makes 15 cubes

There are all sorts of homemade concentrates and purees you can whip up to make your water more festive. But I'm partial to these compound ice cubes. Like its sister citrus, lime juice helps your cells hydrate, and fresh ginger root is an Ayurvedic all-star ingredient with its own long list of medicinal benefits, including as a cure for colds, cramps, and gastrointestinal issues.

....

One 4-inch knob fresh ginger, rinsed and thinly sliced
1 cup (loosely packed) fresh mint leaves, coarsely torn
2 limes, zested and juiced (about $^1/_3$ cup juice)

1. Divide the ginger and mint leaves among the wells of a 15-cube ice tray.

2. Add the lime zest, lime juice, and 1⅔ cups of water to a liquid measuring cup. Stir to combine.

3. Pour the lime mixture into the tray wells. Place in the freezer until solid, about 2 hours. Add a cube to your daily water glass or pitcher, or even to hot tea for a little extra oomph and flavor.

HEALTHY HEDONIST TIPS

Part of the process of eliminating harmful plastics in my home meant replacing my crappy ice cube trays with snazzy, bendable, and easy-to-evacuate silicone models. A generic tray will of course work, but you might need to use two of them to have fifteen 1-ounce slots. I should mention that the square silicone cubes look extra fancy in cocktails and mocktails.

MARKET SWAPS

Fresh basil would be equally delicious in these cubes, as would some diced cucumber for refreshing spa water. If you don't like having the whole leaves in your glass once the ice has melted, you can make an infusion instead. Boil 1⅔ cups of water, then steep the mint and ginger for 20 minutes. Strain through a fine-mesh sieve, stir in the lime juice, and transfer to the ice trays. Another plus of silicone is that you can add hot liquid without worrying about leaching chemicals into your cubes!

"PHO REAL" SLOW COOKER GINGER-CHICKEN BONE BROTH

Makes 2½ to 3 quarts

Many chefs will laugh if you ask how they feel about the bone broth craze. And that's because people have been making slow-cooked stocks since the invention of fire. The longer bones simmer, the more of the marrow, collagen, and gelatin you'll extract from them, which benefits your own bone strength, liver detoxification, and gut lining. This version, inspired by Vietnamese pho, uses fresh ginger and whole spices to make all those immune benefits taste great too. And thanks to modern cooking inventions, you don't even have to mess with fire.

....

1½ pounds chicken bones or 1 pound whole chicken wings

1 pound bone-in chicken thighs

1 large onion, unpeeled and quartered

4 garlic cloves, unpeeled

4-inch knob fresh ginger, sliced

1 tablespoon black peppercorns

1 cinnamon stick

1 tablespoon sea salt

1 jalapeño pepper, halved (optional, if you like heat)

1. Add the chicken bones, chicken thighs, onion, garlic, ginger, peppercorns, cinnamon, salt, and jalapeño (if using) to the bowl of a 6- to 8-quart slow cooker. Cover the ingredients with 4 quarts of water, or enough to submerge them while leaving an inch of room at the top. Cook, covered, on low for 8 hours. Remove the chicken thighs from the broth and shred the meat. Transfer to an airtight container and store for a later use. Return

any skin and bones to the slow cooker and continue cooking for 8 more hours.

2. Over a large bowl or liquid measuring cup, strain the stock through a fine-mesh sieve, discarding the solids once or twice if there's too much pileup.

3. Transfer the bone broth to an airtight container and store in the fridge to sip on throughout the week, freeze in 1-quart servings to cook with, or proceed with the recipe for Vietnamese Chicken Soup for the Soul (page 330).

HEALTHY HEDONIST TIPS

Look for slow cookers that have a stainless steel bowl—some ceramic models can contaminate your food with lead when heated. To make the broth on the stovetop, simply sear the chicken thighs in a pot, followed by the onion, garlic, and ginger. Then add the remaining ingredients. Cook on low heat for 12 hours, removing the chicken thighs and adding more water at the 3-hour mark. If you aren't making Vietnamese Chicken Soup for the Soul (page 330), try combining your shredded chicken with my Coconut Oil–Sriracha Aioli (page 105) and some diced radishes for an Asian spin on chicken salad.

MARKET SWAPS

Like any broth, let this one be a way to use up whatever veggie scraps you have lying around the kitchen. Try adding carrot peelings, fennel fronds, cilantro or mint stems, onion skins, or zucchini tops. Whole star anise would also be a great addition in the spice department.

BACK IT UP

CHIRO-PRACTICAL PHYSICAL THERAPY

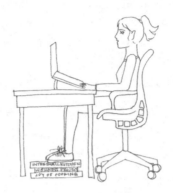

On fortifying my spine and creating habits
for not becoming a hunchback.

I t seemed appropriate that I was starting to reevaluate my work habits just as I approached the halfway mark of my health overhaul.

While most of my experiments were short-term sprints, the whole to-do list still felt very much like a marathon. As I looked back on all of the best practices I'd acquired, I realized how many of them had already begun to slip. It was as if my brain and body could only swallow so many lessons before my stomach rejected them with the fury of a week-old oyster.

In general, my exercise in awareness meant I was paying much more attention to where my spirit stood day in, day out. And I was starting to notice which parts of my wellness equation were still dragging me down—the toxic elements of my life that might be a lot harder to remove than an endocrine-disrupting face wash.

One of those things was how much of my day I spent sitting and the impact that was having on my back.

Having a bad back may not register high on the scale of debili- 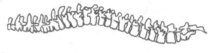 tating illnesses to fear in one's lifetime. But if you look at the numbers, it's clear that our relationship with our faulty spines is a huge piece of the wellness puzzle.

According to a 2011 report from the National Academies of Sciences, Engineering, and Medicine, over one hundred million Americans suffer from chronic pain. That's more than from cancer, heart disease, and diabetes combined. And our bad backs are expensive—everything from surgeries and medications to lost productivity—amounts to about six hundred billion dollars a year.

I've been pretty injury-prone for most of my life, including a rather impressive month in high school during which I managed to tear ligaments in both ankles and then break three toes in my sleep (thanks to a very realistic game of dream soccer). Still, I'd always thought I would at least be the proud owner of a midlife crisis convertible by the time my back decided to go out on me.

Instead, that fateful day came the summer before starting my wellness project as I was preparing to leave for a solo travel adventure in Europe. I wasn't carrying groceries or lifting a heavy skillet—two activities I'd often blamed for my perpetually sore lumbar region. I was simply putting on my pants. And as Miranda Hobbes and I both learned the hard way, throwing out your back is even less fun when you do it while partially naked.

If it hadn't been for the nonrefundable plane ticket, I would have likely stayed belly-up on the floor for hours. Instead, I muscled on my clothes and poured myself into a taxi. On the plane, I pounded Aleve like candy and spent the entire overnight flight pacing up and down the aisle (which didn't thrill the flight attendants). On arrival in Spain, I switched to the local medicine (red wine) to make backpacking with a bad back that much less excruciating.

Painkillers in pill and bottle form got me through the trip, but they were not a long-term solution. Every few months, my back went out again. The severe pain would last for a week, and afterward, I carried around an even more debilitating worry that it was only a matter of time until the next episode.

It was time to finally take a look at the dysfunctional movement patterns that had gotten me into trouble in the first place, one of which I knew was sitting. Reworking my posture would require more thought and effort than purchasing a family-size tub of Bengay or a granny cart for my groceries, but I hoped that by the time I actually was a granny, my new back habits would prevent me from looking like I belonged in the bell tower of Notre Dame.

Sitting Is the New Smoking

There are many things in modern life that can force your spinal alignment out of whack. Wearing high heels pushes your center of balance forward, straining your lower back and causing your calf muscles to shorten, leaving you misaligned when you're walking around barefoot. Driving forces you to favor one side over the other, as do activities like, say, chopping vegetables. But the biggest overall culprit of back, strength, and alignment issues—something that all one hundred million chronically pained Americans might have in common—is sitting.

Over the past few years, "sitting is the new smoking" has become a viral health mantra. The gist is that our increasingly sedentary lifestyle is killing us more than virtually all other man-made poisons and infectious diseases.

For cavemen, life required much more movement. But today our daily routine takes us from bed to chair to car to chair to car to reclining La-Z-Boy. A sweeping study of the health habits of twelve thousand Australian adults found that for every single hour of television watched after the age of twenty-five, the viewer's life expectancy decreased by twenty-two minutes—twice as much as a single cigarette.

Does that make Netflix the new Philip Morris?

Unfortunately, the problem of sitting extends far beyond the couch, and a surgeon general's warning during the opening credits of *Bloodline* is not going to eradicate it anytime soon.

Though I do spend a good amount of time standing over a cutting board, for the rest of the week I sit for a living. I assumed that a moderate exercise habit would counteract some of my sloth-like behavior. But a recent study conducted by Cornell University suggested that the hours spent on our butts are really the prime indicators of mortality, regardless of how many days a week you go to cardio kickboxing before an eight-hour shift at the computer.

When you sit all day, gravity puts enormous pressure on your spine. Being sedentary in a chair also shortens the muscles on the fronts of your hips and the backs of your legs. When we get up, our body continues to subtly hold that unnatural chair-like shape, causing our alignment to shift into a crooked, bowed mess.

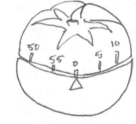

Looking for a rule of thumb to prevent the onset of sitting-related "diseases" didn't turn up any easily applicable consensus. Most extremists recommended I buy a treadmill desk, tatami mat, and Squatty Potty and basically sit never.

The Pomodoro Technique, a productivity system invented by entre-preneur Francesco Cirillo, seemed to offer a happy medium. Cirillo's sys-tem breaks down work into intervals interspersed with short breaks to make larger tasks more manageable. In an effort not to lock myself in that sexy seated C-shape, I would try to get up every forty-five minutes, even if just to walk to the fridge to sneak another spoonful of almond butter.

I set my kitchen timer (sadly, not tomato-shaped like the one that inspired Cirillo's system) to (a) keep me aware of how many minutes I logged in the death grip of my chair and (b) force me to walk to the other side of my studio apartment to turn it off.

I wanted to commit to this "quit sitting" challenge for two weeks, but I knew I couldn't do so without exceptions. If I was out to a long dinner with friends, I wasn't going to go to the bathroom between each course, lest they think I had acquired a urinary tract infection or drug issue since our last shared meal. I decided it was best to deal with this wellness aspect during the workday, on my own time.

Desk-Side Damage Control

By the time I started my project, I had been working from home for over five years.

On most days, I woke up and couldn't believe that people actually paid me to write and cook for a living. With each batch of gluten-free carrot cake pancakes I tested, my time toiling in corporate big beauty seemed more and more distant. And on days when I got to leisurely eat said pancakes in front of an equally indulgent mid-afternoon episode of *House of Cards*, life felt truly sweet.

But despite the flexible hours and occasional workweek TV guilty pleasures, I had started to realize how much I missed my former life of going to an office every day. When you work alone, there's no one there to bounce ideas off of or give you advice in the moment. No one to flash an eye roll if a client is being a pain in the butt or a deal falls through because Mercury is in retrograde. Now that I was alone all day, every day, the absence of community was really starting to weigh on me. Every decision was on my shoulders and every small mistake made me feel like I was destined to still be "faking it 'til I make it" at age forty-five—not to mention never being able to afford that midlife crisis convertible.

As a result, I'd begun noticing an extreme uptick in my neediness. And this, as one can imagine, was not a great thing for my relationship.

While Charlie got to chat with his coworkers all day by the water cooler, by five p.m. I was starved for attention and human contact. If our nighttime plans got derailed because of a last-minute meeting, it felt like a personal affront—proof that he cared more about his career than he did about me.

My sane side recognized these issues for what they were: a product of spending too much time dwelling on my own neurotic, overly analytical thoughts. And I was starting to realize that taking on this project, which forced my wheels of self-analysis into overdrive, might be making matters worse. In fact, it occurred to me one night as I lay awake tossing and turning, my head buzzing with new recipe ideas and fears about that day's dietary missteps, that writing a book about wellness might be one of the unhealthiest things I could ever do to myself.

Besides the self-doubt and isolation, which turned so many of our world's great wordsmiths into terminally depressed alcoholics, the physical ramifications were obvious: it shifted me into a higher sitting gear. These days there were fewer afternoons standing in the kitchen making veggie-packed pancakes and more spent at my desk. When I got on a writing tear, I could lose hours bent over my screen. And on those precious productive occasions, the last thing I needed was an alarm breaking my train of thought every forty-five minutes.

It only took a few days for me to reach my breaking point with the kitchen timer. The loud, startling ring was effective at making me literally jump out of my chair, but it also dissolved my productivity into a puddle of Instagram likes, Vogue.com articles, and texts to my significant other. So much for Mr. Pomodoro's productivity.

I started to look for other ways to make my workplace friendlier for my body, without turning my mind into hostile territory.

Ergonomics 101

Thanks to the emerging field of "inactivity physiology," standing desks are having a moment. And there's accumulating evidence that these workstations have just as much of a positive impact on your head as they do the structure it sits upon.

A group of Canadian researchers analyzed the results of over twenty standing desk studies and found that the majority of participants reported an increase in focus, energy, and happiness, and a decrease in stress and appetite. Similar results were found for the more ambitious treadmill desk, which, as it so happens, was invented by Dr. James Levine, the same guy who coined the phrase "sitting is the new smoking."

Considering I hadn't actually been on a treadmill in years, let alone tried to type while operating one, that option just seemed like another sports-related broken bone waiting to happen. But even if I *had* wanted one, the price tag was prohibitive.

Many companies are starting to invest in workplace wellness benefits, which means that now all of my tech friends in San Francisco have been given the gift of adjustable desktops, in addition to limitless green juice and midday office yoga. But these desks aren't exactly accessible if Google or Dropbox isn't footing the bill.

For we lowly self-employed souls, one cheaper option was an Ikea hack like putting a bookshelf on top of my existing desk. I could see how this might work for people with a lot of surface area to work with, but less so for someone using a hallway console table as a miniature workstation. In addition to the hours I would lose trying to operate my power drill, I worried that this do-it-yourself version would require too large a commitment to standing, since I couldn't switch back to sitting without removing the platform entirely. So I went with the second-cheapest route and, for one hundred dollars, got a manually adjustable riser for my computer and keyboard.

While I waited for the Amazon fairies to deliver my new sit-to-stand podium, I discovered some best practices from ergonomics experts and my standing desk brain trust in Silicon Valley:

1. *Make sure your monitor and keyboard are set at the right height.* It's very easy for people to misuse standing desks and achieve an equally grave hunchback status if they have to look down at their screens. Propping up your monitor or laptop with a stack of books is a good hack if your desk doesn't come with its own adjustable platform. Similarly, your elbows should be at a clean 90-degree angle when your hands rest on the keyboard, so adjust the height accordingly.

2. *Don't stand for long periods of time.* If you get too macho about the standing mission, you risk missing the point. If you stay in the same position for eight hours, it becomes less important that you're sitting versus standing. The idea is to introduce variety and to move.

3. *Choose your intervals wisely.* My friends with standing desks found they weren't able to consistently move the desk up and down several times a day. Rather, they recommended starting the day standing up, when you're at your sleepiest, and then again at the end of the day so you can leave the desk up for the next morning's work session.

4. *Choose your tasks wisely.* I was relieved to learn that most people didn't perform small motor skills at their highest level when forced to

multitask. Studies showed that users of treadmill desks, in particular, suffered some reductions in productivity when doing long periods of typing. It was hard enough for me to churn out articles while sitting, so I knew that my standing time would have to be dedicated to simpler, browsing-oriented activities or responding to emails. And if they devolved into online shopping, I at least would be doing something productive by being on my feet.

IN THE MEANTIME, I also wanted to take my sitting game up a notch by applying some of these same alignment concepts.

The winter after my first back incident, with some help from my parents at Hanukkah, I finally invested in an ergonomic chair whose function was as impressive as its form. I had been using a woven bucket seat, which taught me that what makes for a great Pinterest decor board doesn't always benefit your back. But I realized that I hadn't been taking advantage of my chair's full functionality.

When I checked the 90-degree alignments of my elbows and knees, I noticed that the chair was so low, I looked like a freeze frame from the *Thriller* music video when I typed. If I moved the seat up, though, my legs became overextended. So I put books under my feet to bring my knees back into a 90-degree alignment and then used another stack for my laptop to bring my gaze straight in front of me.

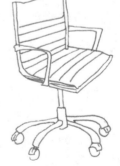

It was a great way to declutter all the cookbooks collecting dust on my windowsills. But it turned my usually tidy workspace into a food-writing Fort Knox.

Back Pain's Back Alright

Even being proactive about my sitting, I still lived in fear that another back episode could happen at any moment. I wasn't entirely convinced that my desk habits were the root cause. After all, at my corporate job I had logged many hours in an ergonomic chair and remained pain-free.

And that fear was validated when my next attack hit.

Somewhere in the middle of taking glamour shots of gluten-free crab cakes, a shooting pain up my right side brought me to my knees so fast, I didn't even have time to worry about the expensive piece of equipment in my hands; my camera and I hit the floor with a thump. Having experienced this before on roughly the same patch of rug, I immediately rolled onto my back and bent my knees to release the tension. Every small movement felt like I was on the receiving end of a Dark Arts unforgivable curse.

To add insult to injury, all of this was happening to a soundtrack of '80s dance hits blasting at a decibel level meant to overpower food processors and sizzling vegetables. I tried to use the music as motivation to reach for my phone that was just four feet away. But Tiffany just didn't have enough oomph to help me fight through the spasms. Eventually, I wedged myself against the coffee table and spent the next hour self-medicating with the crab cakes. In between bites, I pondered my options.

I had already tried the chiropractor route, and while he gave my lifestyle more attention than most standard whack-and-crack operations, his adjustments never seemed to stick. I always ended up reverting to a diverse and ultimately needless array of products and doodads, from drugstore anti-inflammatory creams to earthing biomats (said to limit inflammation by mimicking the naturally healing electric frequencies of the Earth's surface). Most had negligible results and unfortunate side effects that did not appeal to my healthy hedonism. Let's just say a magnetic back brace under high-waisted skinny jeans is not a cute look.

I'd also branched out into other non-chiropractic options during moments of crisis. There was the Alexander Technique, 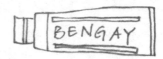 which focused on posture. And of course acupuncture, which I had already been trying with Acu Heidi. She had cupped my back a few times, which temporarily relieved some of the pressure, and left me one Kabbalah bracelet away from looking like a New Age Hollywood celebrity. I had even once called in the big guns of massage: a Rolfer.

"I have two rules," Brian the Body Worker told me. "One, try to relax on the table. And two, don't punch your massage therapist."

After the first five minutes of my session, I had already broken rule number one and was coming dangerously close to breaking number two. Just when I thought Brian's hands had found my most tender trigger point, he would move his finger half an inch to the right and unlock a whole new world of pain. The day after the treatment, my entire back and butt looked like the train of Cruella De Vil's Dalmatian coat, with all the spots roughly the size of Brian's thumbs. His bodywork definitely helped, but as I lay on the floor licking crab cakes off my fingers, I just couldn't bring myself to put my body through the meat grinder again.

Which is how, a few text messages later, I found myself on another massage table across town.

Core Fusion

When I arrived at Juliet Maris's office, I was greeted by a sunny, Winnie Cooper–esque girl next door. I could tell immediately that her approach was different. For every question about my physical history, including illness and injury, Juliet also asked one about my recent emotional state. *Am I the type of person to hold on to things?* Check. *Have I been under a lot of stress at work?* Check check.

We immediately began a series of alignment exercises to see where I was off. And it turned out that I was just as physically crooked as I felt. Juliet noted that my back was curving slightly to the left, yet my right shoulder was lower, causing one hip to jut forward off its axis like a statue of Venus de Milo.

These imbalances were also apparent in my gait. Juliet explained that texting while walking causes people to change their stride completely to compensate for the distraction. Research has shown that these new movement patterns, aside from looking strange, force the body into poor posture, what some refer to as the iHunch. I wondered if my walking habits could have been giving me just as many problems as my sitting habits.

"I need to readjust your pelvis," Juliet said as she helped me onto the table and put some wedges underneath my hips. "You have other misalignments, but when the sacrum is off, we have to fix that first. It affects everything above and below it."

Juliet pressed one hand between my lower back and the table, then gently wiggled my abdomen with the other like she was rolling out a long tube of gnocchi dough.

"So do you think it's my everyday habits that are causing these ongoing issues or a past injury?" I asked, wondering if one of my broken bones in high school had caught up with me.

"Well, if you have an injury that you don't correct through physical therapy, then your whole body is going to compensate and form bad habits on top of it. For you, though, I think the clear problem is a crisis of weakness."

The idea that I was in need of some strengthening exercises didn't come as much of a surprise. After all, in the process of wasting away during the years I binged on gluten, stopped going to the gym, and let my thyroid go untreated, a lot of the weight I'd lost had been muscle mass. I worried, though: how was I supposed to get strong again if every skillet-shaped barbell I lifted felt like it was bringing me to the brink of another back disaster?

Luckily, Juliet told me that traditional exercise wouldn't necessarily address the areas that needed the most attention. When your core isn't stable enough to support itself, even the slightest movements can send your nerve endings into panic mode. And these core problems all stem from the area at the base of the spine: the pelvic floor. This unsung hero of our mid-region provides roots for the whole center body like the base of a tree. And many of our other motor skills and movements (including bowel) rely on it for support.

"I have a client who is super into CrossFit," Juliet told me. "She can do all the really big movements. But her intrinsic muscles—the ones that support posture and balance—are the ones she struggles with. Engaging the more intimate parts of yourself is a totally different process."

As I lay on my back with my hips up on a block in supported bridge pose, Juliet talked me through a sequence to invigorate the inner part of my abdomen.

"Ah . . . so like a Kegel exercise?" I asked.

"No," she replied, clearly having dealt with many a closet *Cosmo* reader. "They are similar, but these go a little deeper. Don't think about holding in your pee but rather pulling the muscle in toward your belly button. Then, you're going to do the same thing with the muscle right below it." I took this to mean the grundle area.

"And finally, engage the anus. We'll just call this one 'number three' so that I don't have to keep saying 'anus.'"

As I silently worked these three muscles one by one, Juliet corrected my pelvis any time it shifted. "There shouldn't be any outward movement. This is all happening internally."

The process was very different from what I had previously thought of as Kegel exercises. It required concentration and focus—not something I could casually do on the subway while listening to Taylor Swift.

Free Your Mind, the Back Will Follow

After a few weeks of Juliet's exercises, I was definitely stronger. Focusing on my pelvic floor made me start to support myself differently. When I went to unload the dishwasher, I engaged my core first to give my back some added protection as I bent down to remove the plates. It was a simple change in awareness that put my spine at ease.

But I still had a lot of tension in my neck and upper back. I had always chalked up my routine aches and pains to my Hashimoto's, which counts muscle soreness and stiffness, especially in the hips and shoulders, among its many symptoms. This tension felt more intense than usual, though. And back on her massage table, Juliet was trying to work it out.

"Do you have any anger?" she asked as she rolled her knuckles into my shoulder blades.

"Anger? Well, yeah. A little bit. Who doesn't?" I replied.

"Is it toward a male figure in your life?"

"Maybe . . ."

"Can you find a way to solve the problem?"

"I don't know."

All of a sudden, I was unfurling a list of Charlie grievances: lack of communication and scheduling quality time in advance, feeling that I was sometimes less important than his job or even his dog. Basically, the signs my fearmongering mind had latched on to that proved this relationship was lopsided, and I better bottle up my vulnerability before I risked getting hurt.

Juliet listened patiently while continuing to knead my neck with her thumbs. "This all makes sense in terms of what I'm feeling," she replied, pulling me from my pity party with her straightforward, soothing tone. "Your tension is all on the right side, which represents the masculine aspects of your personality and any relationship you have with a man. It's also the side associated with the emotion of anger. It's more yang—more aggressive and active. The left side is more yin—feminine, introspective, and intuitive."

"So you think my back problems are because of my feelings toward Charlie?"

"Not all of them. But the more work I do on clients, and the more work I do on myself, I see how so many issues are linked to our emotions. That's what we hold in our bodies."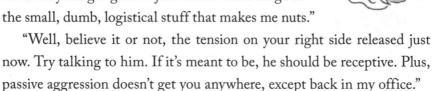

"But what can I do about it? This isn't a toxic relationship. I'm crazy about him, and most of the time everything is great. I just can't seem to let go of the small, dumb, logistical stuff that makes me nuts."

"Well, believe it or not, the tension on your right side released just now. Try talking to him. If it's meant to be, he should be receptive. Plus, passive aggression doesn't get you anywhere, except back in my office."

MANY AUTOIMMUNE SUFFERERS point out emotional, not physical, trigger points as the suspected cause of their disease. And while there's an argument to be made for how our hormones shift from week to week—leaving more room for things to go awry—some have speculated that one reason why thyroid conditions affect three times as many women as men is because of the way we process stress.

"Illness is what happens when women, the nurturers of humanity, forget how to nurture themselves," said Dr. Habib Sadeghi in his TED Talk about how emotions affect our health.

Our words, even those spoken internally, carry weight. And when they attack, isn't it possible that our body is also taught to turn on itself?

There is a particular irony in how Hashimoto's translates that inner dialogue to outward expression; our butterfly-shaped thyroid gland sits on the windpipe below the Adam's apple—our voice box.

"From an emotional and energetic perspective, thyroid dysfunction is a communication disorder," writes Jen Wittman in her book *Healing Hashimoto's Naturally*. In her health coaching practice, Wittman noticed a trend among her clients: they tended to be self-admitted control freaks who avoided conflict and cared deeply about what others thought of them.

"Because we have challenges in expressing ourselves directly, we tend to feel angry or resentful toward others because we cannot confront them and we feel like we don't have a voice," she writes.

I knew, of course, that while I had issues communicating some of my annoyances with Charlie, he wasn't necessarily the root cause of them. My visit with Juliet had forced me to consider how not just the sitting but the daily isolation of being an entrepreneur was affecting my thyroid and my immune system, as well as my sense of self.

I was glad I now had the tools to strengthen my pelvic floor and fortify my spine on my own time. But part of that work was facing how mental tensions were furthering my physical ones. I could never rid my life of stressful situations, but it was within my power to make sure that they didn't show up in my back.

Taming the Tension

When I started researching the emotional side of back pain, I remembered a book that a friend of mine had recommended—one that he credited for helping him return to his job from a back-related medical leave.

In 1973, Dr. John Sarno began his clinical practice at NYU Medical Center for disorders relating to musculoskeletal pain. Conventional medicine had taught him that the cause was structural. But after he grew frustrated by his inability to treat patients successfully using traditional methods, he began noticing a pattern of other tension-related disorders— migraines, irritable bowel syndrome, heartburn, and stomach ulcers— and wondered whether there could be a correlation. Once he shifted his approach from the body to the mind, the results were astonishing. And after years of logging case histories with his new method, Sarno brought his back cure to the masses in his best-selling book.

The crux of *Healing Back Pain* is that unexpressed emotions— particularly anxiety and anger—have physiological consequences that can lead to chronic physical ailments. Anxiety subtly causes shallow breathing. This loss of oxygen to your muscles, tendons, and ligaments builds slowly over time and eventually the tension can add up to an acute attack.

I was a little dubious at first, especially since Sarno's work is still controversial in the mainstream medical community, but as I read my way through the first chapter, I often found myself nodding my head in agreement. Self-critical overachievers, a description very similar to the one I'd read about in *Healing Hashimoto's Naturally*, are particularly prone to tension myositis syndrome (TMS), the official diagnosis Sarno coined for the disorder. Many doctors who don't find a physical issue will tell you it's all in your head. But Sarno's belief is not that your problems are psychosomatic. He recognizes that the pain is very real, it's just being caused by emotional issues, not structural ones.

The treatment plan in *Healing Back Pain* is simple: awareness and understanding. All I had to do to get better was read the book. I also adopted the same mantra that had helped my friend: *I am strong. I am mighty. I feel no pain.*

"Anyone who has had a serious back attack cannot help but live in terror of the next one," says Sarno. "Ironically, by contributing to a high level of anxiety this fear almost guarantees that another attack will come sooner or later."

Like many Californians understand, the longer you have to wait for your fault lines to falter, the greater the fear of the impending Big One. In the case of my back, that fear became a self-fulfilling prophecy—one that left me in a puddle of crab cake crumbs on the floor. My new mantra was a way to make sure my brain was constantly getting a reality check that this attack was never imminent.

Another important part of overcoming this fear is returning to all the intense activities you were doing before your pain started. The physical restrictions these worries breed (perpetuated by medical professionals who tell you not to lift, move, or carry yourself a certain way) are often more debilitating than the pain itself, Sarno writes.

By strengthening my core through Juliet's pelvic-floor exercises, I gained a bit of my confidence back. But if the first part of my back challenge was getting back on my feet, the second part would have to be leaning into my discomfort and fears around more intense physical activity. And that would involve seeing what all the crazy fitness junkies in New York City had been up to all these years.

The Sweet Spot

If sitting is the new smoking, quitting turned out to be just as hard. The loud, startling ring from my kitchen timer every forty-five minutes got really old, really fast. So after a week, I started using another passive technique that harnessed the power of one of my other wellness experiments: hydration.

As it turns out, drinking a lot of water throughout the day pretty much necessitates getting out of your chair once an hour to either (1) refill your glass or (2) go to the bathroom. Continuing to focus on keeping my water bottle full had a great impact on my movement habits and was a whole lot more enjoyable than watching the clock or listening to a loud alarm.

I also learned that, as far as ergonomically friendly workstations go, you get what you pay for. My cheap standing desk sat in my front hallway unopened for a few weeks. And when I finally got around to unwrapping it, true to its price, it was a drag to set up and an even bigger annoyance to move up and down throughout the day.

Heeding the advice of others, I began with just a modest two-hour standing interval in the morning. When I felt myself getting tired toward the end, I noticed that it caused my posture to droop even more than it might have had I been sitting. Standing with bad form (cocking one hip, leaning on a keyboard tray) can be just as bad for your back as sitting. After a week of use, I decided I'd rather find other creative ways to improve my workspace and promptly sold my standing desk platform on Craigslist.

The easiest change was simply raising my computer screen. Having my laptop straight out in front of my face seemed to have the biggest improvement on my posture. It allowed my shoulders to drop and gave my neck a temporary break from iHunch. Eventually, I dismantled my cookbook towers and invested in a thirty-dollar laptop stand.

Since I was still sitting for my typing work, I started taking my phone calls while standing. Once I learned not to pace into areas of my apartment where the reception dropped, I found that moving while talking kept my train of thought clearer and prevented me from the temptation of reading emails while maintaining a conversation on the other line.

These desk-side strategies were great for maintenance—for not getting into trouble in the first place. But for someone already experiencing chronic back pain, they felt a little like the equivalent of polishing a pair of shoes that already had a hole in the sole. Eventually, I had to take my body to the cobbler to address some foundational issues.

IF YOUR ALIGNMENT is off, that's the first thing that needs to be fixed. But if you don't have a strong core, there's nothing to prevent your sacrum from shifting right back out of place after an adjustment. I learned this the hard way before my project started, after a few failed chiropractor visits. My lower body had become too insecure to stabilize itself, so it used scare tactics to try to get me to move as little as possible.

Once I got some strength back with my morning pelvic-floor exercises, I began to ease into a Pilates practice—first with an app that gave me a ten-minute sequence to do on my floor in the mornings, and then with a more intense weekly mat class at a local studio. Yoga had sometimes caused me more pain as I tried to bend myself into positions that were beyond the scope of my rickety spine. But the slow and targeted movements in Pilates helped isolate problem areas and rehabilitate them.

After a month of Pilates and pelvic-floor exercises, I could get away with some of my bad writing habits without feeling that dull worrying pain. And keeping my back mantra in mind reminded me that another episode was not necessarily brewing in the background.

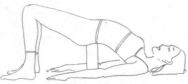

It also made me realize that I had bigger office issues than just my desk posture.

So even though the chairs were wobbly and non-ergonomic, I tried to relocate to a coffee shop for part of the week and make co-working dates with fellow self-employed friends. The setup may not have been as good for my alignment, but getting out of isolation was a big boon to my spirit, even if the only conversation I had was with the person taking my tea order. And when my day included more human contact, it put much less pressure on Charlie to rescue me from my food-writing Fort Knox.

Healthy Hedonist Back Tips

While it's worth tackling the bigger issues first (alignment, core strength, stress), here are some other best practices that can help you heal without a professional and limit muscle imbalances in the first place.

1. *Take calls while standing up or pacing.* Stanford researchers who studied creativity found that sitting is the better option when you have to solve a problem for which there is only one right answer, but walking allowed people to come up with more unique ideas. We don't all have Steve Jobs's status, so forcing your colleagues to attend meetings on a walking trail is probably not realistic. The phone is a nice middle ground. The person on the other end never needs to know you're doing squats while listening to their status report.

2. *Don't favor one side.* Everyone tends to use one side of the body more than the other for simple tasks like carrying a purse, steering a car, brushing your teeth, or talking on a cell phone. Try using your less dominant arm whenever possible. Yoga puts a lot of emphasis on this symmetry. It helps keep the brain and body balanced when you make an extra effort to use your more vulnerable side. Also, consider swapping your tote or purse for a backpack— the load is distributed more evenly, which makes it a better option than a bag that pulls on one side.

3. *Put your load on wheels.* Don't let memories of kids with rolling backpacks getting bullied in the school yard dissuade you from using some of their adult equivalents. You should have no shame

using a granny cart instead of a canvas tote for groceries or a far less chic roll-on suitcase instead of a heavy leather shoulder bag. If you're going on a trip, why not let your back take a vacation too?

4. *Buy an ergonomic chair.* You spend a lot of time in this puppy every single day, so it's worth investing in a good one. The more adjustability, the better—moving the armrests, seat depth, and height will help you achieve the right angles at your workstation. Also, choose a chair with wheels so you can easily get closer and farther away from the computer.

5. *Start and end your day with a desk stretch.* Not only does a set of stretches force you to change position, but it also reminds you to slow down and take a few deep, healing belly breaths, which is equally important for preventing back pain. Try a forward fold over your legs, a simple spinal twist, or a runner's lunge. Consider this your five-minute warm-up lap for your sitting marathon and then a way to release some of the tension at the end of the race.

6. *Sleep on your back.* When it comes to physical recovery, there's a clear hierarchy in sleep positions. Stomach sleepers have it the worst. If you sleep facedown, gravity causes your spine to bow and torques your neck in one direction, even more so if you have a soft mattress. Sleeping on your side is slightly better, especially if you place a pillow between your legs. But the best position for your alignment is sleeping on your back. Put a pillow or a bolster underneath your knees and relax your arms by your sides, or rest them on your stomach.

7. *Limit high heels.* As a woman, I know it's not realistic or culturally acceptable to wear orthopedic shoes to da club. But we could all probably benefit from limiting high heels to more targeted occasions. Not only are they hard on your poor feet, but they strain

your lower back. If you wear heels at the office, try switching to flats when you're sitting at your desk and during your commute.

8. *Strengthen your feet.* A lot of people invest in expensive orthotics for support when they should really be building a better foundation for their feet. Walk barefoot as much as possible. If you're standing, try lifting your toes and applying different pressures to your heel. Your feet are the web of joints that keep you sailing through life. Strengthening them will only improve your balance and stability.

9. *Move with soft knees.* Locking your knees reduces blood flow to your legs and causes your muscles to tighten. When you stand, try making a subtle adjustment and allow your knees to be soft, keeping a slight bend at the joint. This is something you can do when walking and exercising too. You don't need to look like a surfer—the change should be so small that no one will notice.

10. *Use tennis balls for an at-home massage.* Hiring someone to relieve your tension can be very therapeutic. But if you can't afford to get massages on a regular basis (and who can, really?), pick up a can of tennis balls and let them make sweet love to your trigger points. You can lean up against a wall or, for more intensity, lie on the floor. Putting two balls inside a long sock will help you get symmetrical back massage action on both sides of your spine. Rolling your feet on a ball is another way to get them to fall back in love with you or replace a significant other who's not that into foot rubs.

GOLDEN MILK CHIA PUDDING WITH CINNAMON YOGURT

Serves 4

As you know, color is a great indicator of anti-inflammatory properties. And few foods are more vibrant and medicinally powerful than turmeric. If you're feeling achy and inflamed, add a little medicine from your spice rack instead of popping a painkiller. Make a batch of this golden milk pudding to enjoy before your first shift at your desk—it's basically Ayurvedic Advil added to an already wholesome jar of super seeds.

....

Two 15-ounce cans full-fat coconut milk (4 cups)

3 tablespoons pure maple syrup

1 teaspoon vanilla extract

$3/4$ teaspoon ground turmeric

$1/2$ teaspoon ground cinnamon

$1/8$ teaspoon ground ginger

$1/3$ cup chia seeds

$3/4$ cup plain full-fat Greek yogurt (about one 7-ounce container)

1. In a medium saucepan set over medium heat, combine the coconut milk, 1 tablespoon maple syrup, the vanilla, turmeric, ¼ teaspoon cinnamon, and the ginger. Bring to a simmer, whisking until the spices are well incorporated and the milk is a vibrant golden hue, about 2 minutes. Be careful that the milk doesn't boil over! Transfer the golden milk to a mixing bowl and chill in the fridge, covered, until room temperature, about 20 minutes.

2. Add the chia seeds to the golden milk, stirring to distribute. Cover and refrigerate until the chia seeds are plumped, at least 3 hours or overnight.

3. Meanwhile, stir together the yogurt, the remaining 2 tablespoons maple syrup, and the remaining ¼ teaspoon cinnamon in a small mixing bowl until smooth. Cover and set aside in the fridge.

4. Stir the pudding to make sure there are no clumps, then spoon into individual bowls, 8-ounce mason jars, or ramekins (about ¾ cup per container). Add 2 heaping tablespoons of the cinnamon yogurt and enjoy. The premade chia pudding cups will keep, refrigerated, for up to 4 days.

HEALTHY HEDONIST TIPS

The recipes in this book are intentionally low in sugar, but since the flavor of turmeric can be intense for spice newbies, a little maple syrup in the golden milk helps. The cinnamon yogurt is on the sweeter side. As you get more used to the tangy flavor of yogurt and the savory nature of the pudding's spices, you can reduce the maple syrup to 1 tablespoon.

MARKET SWAPS

To make this recipe vegan, you can use coconut cream instead of yogurt. Whisk vigorously (preferably with an eggbeater) to get it thick and frothy before adding in the sweetener and spices.

TURMERIC-BRAISED CHICKEN LEGS WITH GOLDEN BEETS AND LEEKS

Serves 4

One dish that I riff on again and again during my weekend batch-cooking sessions is a Moroccan tagine. The stew is layered with spices and is perfect for making cheaper cuts of meat tender. One weekend afternoon when I had a few pans going on the stovetop, I decided to create an oven-roasted version with whole chicken legs, a bunch of baby golden beets, and sliced leeks. It's super hands-off: you simply toss all the ingredients together in a casserole dish, douse it with white wine, and forget about it in the oven until the chicken skin is browned and the beets and turmeric have created a rich, golden broth that will make you want to lick the bowl. I like to serve the chicken and veggies over quinoa or mashed sweet potatoes.

....

2 leeks, white and light green parts only

1 bunch of golden beets with their greens, scrubbed

2 garlic cloves, minced

2 teaspoons ground turmeric

1 teaspoon ground ginger

1^1/$_2$ teaspoons sea salt

^{1}/$_4$ cup freshly squeezed lemon juice

^{1}/$_4$ cup olive oil

2 pounds whole chicken legs

^{1}/$_2$ cup white wine

1. Preheat the oven to 425°F.

2. Slice the leeks in half lengthwise. Rinse them, fanning out the outer layers to wash away any grit. Slice the cleaned leeks into thin half-moons.

3. Remove the greens from the beets. Rinse them and coarsely chop. Halve the beets and cut each section into four wedges.

4. In a large mixing bowl, toss the leeks, beets, and beet greens together with the garlic, turmeric, ginger, salt, lemon juice, and olive oil until thoroughly combined. Spoon the mixture into a 9 x 13-inch baking dish or casserole pan and arrange in an even layer.

5. Add the chicken to the mixing bowl and toss to coat in the remaining turmeric mixture. Transfer the chicken legs to the baking dish and nestle in the beet mixture. Drizzle any of the remaining marinade over the top of the chicken and pour the wine around the sides of the dish.

6. Roast, uncovered, until the chicken is fork-tender and the beets are soft, about 1 hour.

HEALTHY HEDONIST TIPS

Whole chicken legs will be the most affordable option, as they require less labor at the butcher counter. But you can sub boneless, skinless thighs if you like. It's no longer the '90s, so we don't have to feel bad about eating dark meat or chicken skin. And thank goodness for that, because the added fat helps keep the meat juicy during extended stays in the oven.

MARKET SWAPS

Choose beets that are on the smaller side, about 2 inches in diameter. If you can't find the golden variety, try using a bunch of radishes or baby turnips with their greens instead. Red beets will create a very different final presentation—their color is intense! Scallions, ramps, and shallots will work in place of the leeks, or you can add a mix of all of the above for a vegetarian version.

MAKING MOVES

FITTING FITNESS INTO EVERYDAY LIFE

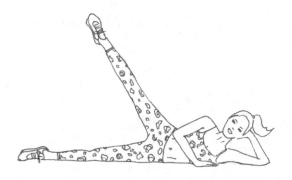

On hitting the pavement and making exercise
into something enjoyable.

The crisis of weakness I discovered during my back challenge didn't happen overnight. My fitness level had been slowly unraveling ever since my Hashimoto's diagnosis.

Back in high school, I was always moving. When it wasn't organized sports, I was doing roundhouse kicks to a Billy Blanks DVD in my living room, running outside to the beat of Destiny's Child, or going to yoga classes with my dad. During college, the frequency diminished and soundtracks changed, but the activities stayed relatively the same. In my early twenties, I could go a month without exercising and then snap my quads back into gear with a four-mile run. But when those months turned into years, I eventually reached a point before starting this project when I realized I had officially "let myself go."

What kicked off this cardio nosedive in the first place was that every time I tried to run, I would get a horrible pelvic cramp within minutes. The culprit? A lasagna brick of gluten lodged in my intestines.

Though my stomach issues had been corrected for the most part, I had replaced one physical barrier with another: the fear around my spine, which had turned even gentle practices like yoga into a once-a-month affair. It was high time I started using my weaknesses as a reason to get strong again, instead of as an excuse not to exercise. After all, it was this loss of muscle mass—and stress—more so than my daily desk habits that had gotten me into trouble with my back in the first place. And the one thing that's best known to combat both is movement.

DURING THE HEIGHT of my college fitness, I used to think about exercise mainly in terms of shedding pounds and getting rid of my muffin top before spring break. It turns out, though, that weight loss is one of the least documented benefits of exercise. Rather, the better argument for getting in shape is to prevent disease in the long term and increase focus, productivity, and happiness in the short term.

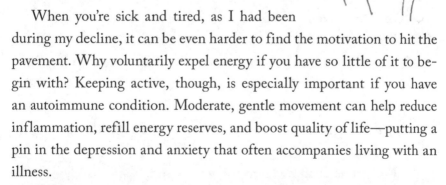

When you're sick and tired, as I had been during my decline, it can be even harder to find the motivation to hit the pavement. Why voluntarily expel energy if you have so little of it to begin with? Keeping active, though, is especially important if you have an autoimmune condition. Moderate, gentle movement can help reduce inflammation, refill energy reserves, and boost quality of life—putting a pin in the depression and anxiety that often accompanies living with an illness.

Antidepressants are some of the most widely prescribed medications for Hashimoto's sufferers, as hypothyroidism can negatively affect dopamine and serotonin levels. And after confronting some of these feelings during my back challenge, I knew that adding some natural opioids to my life through moving more every day couldn't hurt.

But I also felt slightly paralyzed by what "real" exercise required. When most of your friends spend their off-work hours shocking their bodies into shape with resistance bands, free weights, and treadmill sprints at Barry's Bootcamp, it can make going to Pilates once a week or spending eight minutes with an abs app in your living room feel like the bare minimum.

For my next experiment, I wanted to see if pushing myself outside my fitness comfort zone would yield more of those endorphins I was after. And since I was already doing the bare minimum, I wanted to figure out the easiest, healthiest, and most sustainable ways I could make more moves without spending half my rent money on neon leggings and Soul-Cycle classes.

Getting Your Movement Nutrients

No one can really argue with exercise. Like eating your vegetables, it's a pretty universally accepted part of a balanced, healthy life. But there's still a lot of debate over how much is actually necessary to get the job done. And a few recent studies suggest that we non–gym rats might actually be doing better than we think.

During the few occasions that I actually made time for movement, the "runs" I would go on were mostly aspirational: I would get so winded after just one block that I needed to take a walking break. Eventually I just started saying I was going for a walk-run, since the running ratio was too low to justify top billing.

As I began researching exercise intensity and ideal time input, I discovered that this sad fitness program did have some merit. "Wogging," as it's known, is recommended for people who want to develop a running habit but don't yet have the muscular strength or endurance. The idea of switching between more aggressive movement and resting periods is also central to the burgeoning fitness trend of high-intensity interval training, or HIIT.

Researchers have found that pushing your body for a very short period of time—thirty to sixty seconds—and then rewarding your efforts with a comparable session of recovery is much more effective at improving cardiovascular function, building muscle, and burning body fat than longer sustained periods of moderate exercise.

The explanation for why this works dates back to our Paleo forefathers. In the bush, the impulse to run mainly revolved around hunting or being hunted. There was no light jogging while roaming the plains for food, let alone for recreation. Energy was a scarce resource and needed to be conserved for times when quick movement was actually necessary, like escaping a lion or pouncing on your own target.

Even during more intense intervals, my wogging clearly never rivaled the speed needed to flee a big cat. But I liked the idea that these intense periods of exercise need not exceed the time it would take either to outwit or to be eaten by 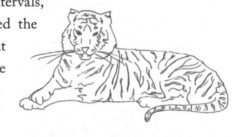 one. In fact, HIIT's biggest appeal is that the regimen uses your time efficiently. The suggested protocol is one twenty-minute session, three times a week.

Time-wise, that seemed rather doable. But efficiency bonus points aside, other research suggested that intensity plays a smaller role. Recently, several sprawling studies have uncovered the ideal exercise dose for a longer life: 150 minutes a week, 30 minutes of that being vigorous. That means that outside of your half-hour go-big-or-go-home phase, simply strolling could be enough to ward off premature death.

Walking might seem like a lame form of exercise. But it's also a biological imperative, perhaps even more important for survival in this modern life of ours than learning to sprint away from a hypothetical animal of prey.

"Exercise is movement, but movement is not always exercise," writes Katy Bowman in her book *Move Your DNA: Restore Your Health Through Natural Movement.* "And exercise does not always make every part of us better." Just as our diet benefits from containing as many different nutrients as possible, Bowman argues that our bodies need a variety of different "loads" placed on it to fuel our musculoskeletal fitness—which she believes is much more important than our cardiovascular system.

And what's the movement equivalent of a bowl of kale? Walking.

Especially when done naturally—meaning, on a varied terrain—walking uses a greater number of muscles than most other activities. Running on a treadmill may get oxygen flowing, but it's the same movement over and over again. It has a very limited load profile and, therefore, not many movement nutrients. It's a salad at TGI Friday's, while walking is like taking your cells out to eat at Gwyneth Paltrow's house.

So to begin my foray into getting my body back in shape, I decided to forget the gym membership and HIIT and just focus on moving for at least thirty minutes every day. My moderate movement goal probably wouldn't give me Barry's abs, but it seemed like a less terrifying place to start than sprinting to the drugstore or doing burpees to the beat of a Katy Perry remix.

Step by Step, Day by Day

During my first week of more movement, I felt like I was getting my thirty minutes in by choosing the less lazy commute. Instead of taking the subway a few stops, I'd leave a little earlier and walk. Instead of the elevator, I'd take the stairs. Instead of hailing a cab, I'd hop on one of the city's bike shares (and then try not to get hit by that forgone cab while riding it).

But was this enough?

One of the things I'd struggled with so far on my wellness journey was the lack of hard data. I had Dr. A's quarterly blood work to give me some clues into how my body was functioning. But it was hard to know if wearing less toxic makeup, drinking more water, and eliminating the chlorine from my shower was really making the long-term difference I felt it was on a cellular level. Could the improvements in energy be a placebo effect? As I learned during back health month, the mind can sometimes be our best and worst medicine.

In terms of learning to tune in to my body, having to rely on subjective assessments was a good thing. But this month, I found myself craving real numbers to crunch—besides just the ones on a scale.

Luckily, fitness arm candy has become as popular today as slap bracelets were in the '80s. So I turned to this new world of wearable tracking devices to tell me if I was doing as well or as poorly as I thought I was.

Gretchen Rubin, the doyenne of happiness, believes that monitoring is one of the pillar strategies for change. As she writes in her book *Better Than Before: Mastering the Habits of Our Everyday Lives*, "self-measurement brings self-awareness, and self-awareness strengthens our self-control." Numbers can be a helpful way of holding up a mirror to our own behavior. In health surveys, people tend to overestimate their physical activity and underestimate their food intake. But with a tracker for accountability, it's harder to delude yourself. As a result, researchers at Stanford University School of Medicine found that wearing pedometers encouraged sedentary people to increase their physical activity significantly.

While they take the subjectivity out of your health equation, trackers also appeal to the ego. It's inspiring to see your progress and perhaps even more so to see it as compared to that of your mother, brother, or significant other. Competition can be as powerful a motivator as a new bandage dress, upcoming trip to the Bahamas, or a chance encounter with an ex.

I wasn't sure I wanted to engage Charlie's competitive spirit; just bringing up the prospect of dueling trackers launched a heated debate over whose legs were longer and how that should be accounted for. But I was still interested to see how my thirty minutes of movement stacked up to the standard benchmark of ten thousand steps a day. So I ordered a neon pink Jawbone UP band that Kelly Kapowski would have been proud of and slapped it on my wrist.

The Road Less Traveled

After two weeks of step tracking, it became apparent that my own internal estimations had been way off. The afternoons I took a thirty-minute walk and sat on my butt writing for the rest of the day, I didn't come even close to ten thousand steps. On the other hand, when I was out on the town pounding the pavement between meetings, I racked up steps easily. In fact, my single highest day involved no official exercise, just a night of bouncing up and down singing '80s karaoke.

My steps in the kitchen, though, scored far below what I had imagined. Even the rigorous hours of de-stemming kale and mincing garlic during my weekend batch-cooking session didn't appear to be an adequate substitute for a walk. This was a letdown, considering how exhausted I always felt afterward.

According to Dr. Nate Meckes, who studied the accuracy of fitness trackers across a variety of movements, one of the issues with these devices is that they don't adequately record subtle standing activities like sweeping and cleaning. For brisk walking on a flat surface, they perform well. But their inability to account for different types of activities, he said, could discourage people from seeking them out. According to the

Harvard School of Public Health, chores do in fact reap a significant physical reward. Vacuuming, mowing the lawn, and other vigorous housework are classified as moderate-intensity exercise. Perhaps rinsing a dish wouldn't get my heartrate up to between 110 and 140 beats per minute, but scrubbing my heavy cast-iron skillet did count for something, even if my wristband didn't think so.

Another issue with fitness trackers is that they don't reflect the fact that not every step is created equal. From a musculoskeletal fitness perspective, fifty steps on a treadmill is very different from fifty steps on the side of a mountain, or even fifty steps pushing a vacuum around your living room. And taking those steps in shoes is very different from doing so barefoot. This all has to do with Katy Bowman's load philosophy, which is echoed by fellow barefoot running enthusiast Christopher Mc-Dougall. In his book *Natural Born Heroes*, McDougall talks about the benefits of exercising in nature, where uncertain paths force you to be nimble and in the moment rather than treating your body like a mindless machine.

Both Bowman and McDougall argue that our modern preference for choosing the cushy road most traveled has contributed to our pervasive weakness. For our ancestors, gaining size and muscle mass was never the goal. Rather, survival depended on being agile. The same can even be said of our forefathers just a few generations ago working the land or scrubbing the floor.

One recent study tested the importance of musculoskeletal fitness by seeing how well participants could get up off the floor from a seated position. Those who could perform the movement without using their hands, or even using just one, were more likely to live longer than those who couldn't. The research indicated that high levels of flexibility and coordination are better indicators of our long-term survival than aerobic fitness.

As kids, we spent a lot of time on the floor. As adults, we can barely sit cross-legged for long enough to make it through a round of Duck Duck Goose, let alone get up once tagged. After passing the floor test with modest results, I knew I had to do more to diversify my movement patterns so I was getting as many loads as possible. Cooking was a bigger plus than my tracker led me to believe, but there also 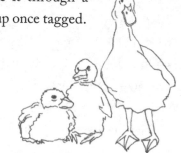 seemed to be an argument for those squat thrusts, burpees, and other movements I could never imagine doing unless someone was making me.

A Class Above the Rest

My fears around organized fitness may have been just as much mental as physical.

The exhaustion and weakness I felt over the years of hypothyroid flare-ups had slowly lowered my expectations of what I was capable of. When I saw friends training for marathons, I knew that such an athletic feat was not within the realm of possibility for me. I was the girl for whom a day of standing in the kitchen felt like exercise. The girl who felt like she had run a marathon simply by switching trains at Times Square in the swampy summer heat. But my daily thirty-minute walks were beginning to remind me what movement could do for my mind, especially when I left my phone at home. After a few weeks of prioritizing these work breaks, I found myself returning to my desk feeling focused and uplifted.

I realized that Sarno's argument for pushing myself further went beyond the scope of my back health: taking on more rigorous physical challenges was also what I needed to push past other mental limitations caused by my disease. I didn't just have to return to the yoga and wogging that predated my first back attack. I needed to get back to the more intense workouts I was doing before I got sick in the first place.

The fitness world had changed considerably since my last gym membership lapsed, which only fueled my fears of not being able to keep up physically. Instructors have been elevated to Hollywood celebrity status, thanks in part to the big-name Hollywood celebrities who swear by them for getting Hervé Léger–ready heinies, and trendy workout devotees flock from one boutique studio to the next.

The epitome of cult exercise—and the first circle of hell in terms of my fitness terror—was SoulCycle. Friends of mine referred to their relationship with the forty-five-minute stationary bike dance party as an addiction. With its steamy club-like atmosphere and homegrown brand of motivational speaking, SoulCycle appealed to them as much more than just a good workout. There was the joy of riding to curated hip-hop or the soundtrack of *Rent*, the choreographed dance moves, the room of familiar faces suffering through the workout with them. As one friend opined, "Sometimes you're too tired to carry yourself. You need the energy in the room to pull you through, in life and in spin class."

For many, all of this is well worth the price of admission. For others, the price of admission justifies itself; prepaying for fitness classes ensures you'll actually haul ass to the studio so you don't lose your money. There was a good six months that I aspirationally maintained a gym membership without going even once. Perhaps prepaying for a specific experience would be a more efficient way to spend my money, even if I wasn't entirely convinced that the experience itself—getting misted by pseudo-spirituality and sweaty twentysomethings—was my cup of tea.

In order to switch up my movement routine, break through my autoimmune barriers, and attempt to find a boutique spinning shoe that fit, I resolved to try at least two new classes a week. I signed up for ClassPass, an app that gave me onetime monthly access to the best studios in my city's backyard for less than I would spend on individual sessions. With the fitness world having exploded, hopefully that meant there really was something out there for everyone, even an exercise Goldilocks like myself.

Buddy System

As much as I wanted to dive in head and untoned arms first, I wasn't quite sure where to start. Reading snarky articles in *New York Magazine* about the latest trends was very different from actually knowing what to expect once I was in the room.

One of the things that had kept me from embracing group exercise classes was that I hate feeling like a newbie. Even trying a different yoga studio gives me mild anxiety. The idea of shadowboxing or pole dancing, where I wouldn't even be familiar with the general movements, let alone the studio layout, was particularly daunting. I may have previously rolled my eyes at fitness cult followers, but in some ways I understood it. Being a regular has many perks, from having the dance routines reinforced through muscle memory to simply knowing how to program the security code on your locker.

I wanted to become part of a community. I just didn't know which calorie-free Kool-Aid to sample first. I needed guidance, a fitness sensei to show me the ropes.

Research has shown that finding a workout buddy can be extremely effective in improving your fitness.

Part of this is accountability. One study revealed that simply receiving a check-in call asking about your exercise progress every two weeks was enough to boost individuals' performance. But the second factor, again, has to do with ego. Just like comparing scores on a fitness tracker or the leader board of a Flywheel spin class, no one wants to be the weakest link, either in a group setting or a one-on-one scenario. Working out with someone who is in slightly better shape than you tends to be the best thing to kick your ass into the next gear.

I considered and rejected the idea of making Charlie my workout buddy, since he and I were already sadly engaged in an informal competition for the *least* amount of time spent exercising. His schedule wouldn't have been conducive to joint fitness sessions anyway. Instead, I warily reached out to a friend who also worked from home and might have time to attend classes during off-peak hours.

"OMG, I thought you'd never ask!" Sarah exclaimed when I posed the question to her over vodka gimlets and expensive salads. Her enthusiasm was reassuring, but I still worried that her fitness level would be too extreme for my taxed adrenals and mushy physique.

"Don't get too excited," I said. "You're going to be doing a lot of hand-holding. But hopefully taking my SoulCycle virginity will be worth it?"

"I would be honored to take it," she said, taking a pause between bites of heirloom radishes. "The only thing is, I don't really do spin anymore."

"Really?" I asked, surprised. "I thought you were the reigning queen of Flywheel."

"That I was! But it just doesn't get my heart rate going anymore."

While she waited for her name to get moved to the top of Tracy Anderson's two-year wait list, Sarah told me she had started going exclusively to a new studio called SLT.

"It's just like Pilates, but way harder," she gushed.

I didn't find this terribly encouraging, but at least I had some prior experience with Pilates. I committed to my first advance booking right there at the table. It cost the same as the tab for my kale Caesar and Kettle One.

Megaforming My Body

When I arrived at class the following week, it became immediately apparent that what I thought of as Pilates was very different from what I was about to experience. The "MEGA heart-pumping, muscle-quivering workout" advertised on the website appeared to be taking place exclusively in the carriage of a Megaformer, a traditional Pilates machine on steroids, or something you might find in Christian Grey's sex dungeon.

I sat by the front desk watching an earlier class finish. The room was full, which left me wondering: who were all these fembots doing oblique curls at ten thirty a.m. on a Monday?

When Sarah arrived she must have seen the look of dread on my face as I watched the Amazonian women hurl themselves back and forth on their carriages. (It was the cool-down portion.)

"Don't worry!" she reassured me. "You can rest in child's pose whenever you need to. I always do."

When the turnover came, we made our way to neighboring machines and the teacher came over to introduce herself. She showed me how to adjust the straps and springs, and as she explained which color coordinated with which weight, I got the same mild headache that I get while shopping at Ikea.

After five minutes, the muscle quivering kicked in for my legs, which made my relationship with the Megaformer that much more precarious. I spent most of the hour just trying not to slip on my own sweat and careen off of it.

"How do you feel?!" Sarah asked me afterward, dabbing small beads of sweat from her brow, her blond hair still perfectly straight and wisp-less.

"Humbled," I replied, making no effort to hide my defeat. While everyone else was plowing through the routines with their beach bods, I had been flopping around like a beached fish.

"Oh stop! You did so well."

"Do you see my machine?" I said, pointing at the bench. "It looks like the front row at SeaWorld."

"Isn't it great? You sweat so much—that's what makes it such a good workout!"

For the record, she did not rest in child's pose once.

Feel the Burn

The next day, I could barely walk. Every time I laughed my stomach muscles responded with their own swan song of anguish. I required much more than two hands to get up from the floor; I felt like I needed a forklift just to sit on the toilet. Not a good sign for my musculoskeletal well-being.

That weekend, I accompanied a group of friends—all wearing matching purple bachelorette tank tops—to 305 Fitness for an eight a.m. hip-hop class. Ordinarily, this would have been the portion of the girls' weekend festivities that I skipped. As the DJ dropped his first beat and the whole room began twerking in unison, I immediately regretted my choice.

It was another sobering experience, combining the two physical activities I had begun to fear most: coordinated dance and cardio. Ten minutes in, I accidentally turned the wrong way and gave the bride an enthusiastic whip to her nae nae. Soon thereafter, I peeled off to the side to mop my face and observe the more coordinated masses from a comfortable distance, but the Taye Diggs look-alike in charge was having none of that. He shimmied to the corner, grabbed my hand, and grinded me back to the center of the room.

The following week, still feeling the burn from getting my body rocked on the dance floor and in the carriage of my Megaformer, I chose a class I hoped would be slightly less brutal because most of the action would be taking place in the air.

Light, daily bouncing on a personal trampoline is one of the many wacky prac- 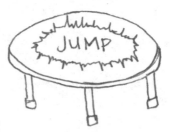 tices recommended for people who suffer from thyroid disorders. Since I didn't have room for a rebounder in my studio apart- ment, I was excited to find a studio that would give me the opportunity to stimulate my lymphatic system and get my blood pumping in a group setting.

Bouncing might have been low impact, but the version I experienced at Bari wasn't necessarily a salve to my heart. As I jumped higher and higher, it became harder and harder to keep up with the dance routines (which were now airborne). After I came dangerously close to landing wrong on my ankle, I decided to sit the last ten minutes out. Not even a pep talk from Béla Károlyi could get me back on my apparatus.

THE FOLLOWING WEEKS included spinning, barre method, pole dancing, cardio yoga, and a mash-up workout at the decidedly apropos "The Class."

The hour was a mix of interval training and aerobic mat work, combined with emotional catharsis. And the latter was achieved by encouraging us to break through psychological barriers by yelling at the top of our lungs. As I balanced in plank pose, women wailing all around me, I wished they had included free earplugs at the check-in counter as they had at the cardio dance class the week prior.

Like the warm-up act at a self-help conference, the instructor asked probing questions into her wireless mic. *What in your life is standing in your way? What parts of yourself do you want to get unstuck?*

"Come on. Let it all out!" Cue banshee screaming.

I was all for self-reflection and breaking down the walls that were holding me back. I just didn't necessarily want to be doing those things in between jumping jacks.

When someone is talking to you about changing your life in the context of squat thrusts, it's hard not to see that change as being related to your imperfect physique. Sure, for many women in the room, losing weight was the main reason they were there. But this line of inspiration just felt off. There was a lot of emphasis on looking within yourself but not a whole lot about listening to your body.

People these days—especially New Yorkers—are incredibly focused on maximizing their time, and each fitness class I tried catered to that compulsion. There was seldom talk of modifying postures if I was having trouble—it was all about pushing through the pain. And in the name of efficiency, so few of them took time away from the heart-pumping exercise to help me wind down properly at the end. Not only did I feel like this wasn't doing my limbs any favors, but I could tell my adrenals were in shock. I ended up going to bed at nine thirty p.m. on some workout days. I slept great, one of the benefits of exercise, but the fatigue and muscle pain lasted the whole week.

I also noticed how the financial incentive could push you too far. At expensive workouts, there's a feeling that you have to get your money's worth, to complete as many reps and burn as many calories as possible to make the experience worthwhile. But this can do more harm than good, especially when it ignites your fight-or-flight response.

"If you feel like crap after a long run or a spin class, your body isn't just being annoying. It's telling you that it needs rest," says functional medicine entrepreneur Dr. Robin Berzin. "I find that a lot of my clients, especially in their busy city lives, are depleted. They need to restore more than they need to sweat everything out. When you're in that state—where your blood sugar is low and your cortisol spikes—then you can actually perpetuate stress."

In fact, research has shown that the results you're after at the gym—toning, strengthening, pound shedding—are actually easier to achieve if you let your body take a break.

One Danish study pitted two groups of sedentary folks against each other, with one doing twice as much cardio each week as the other. The group that burned half the calories ended up losing more weight than the high-intensity group. The assumption was that the moderate exercisers had more time to recover, and therefore more energy to propel them through the week. They also had less of the surge in appetite that, coupled with exhaustion, left me starfished on the couch after inhaling half my body weight in pasta by the end of week one.

Another downside of all the muscle-quivering exercise was that I found myself back on the take-out train more than once. It was all too easy to rationalize a gluttonous meal as a reward for all my sweat hours logged. This type of justification is called moral licensing. According to Kelly McGonigal, author of *The Willpower Instinct*, giving yourself permission to do something "bad" (e.g., eating pad Thai and watching five straight hours of *The Real Housewives*) because you've been so "good" (e.g., going to SLT) is the kind of mentality that sabotages goals, she writes.

But I was also too tired to make better choices. Hauling ass home after an intense workout, I just didn't have the strength to stand in the kitchen and prepare dinner from scratch. Even pressing defrost on the microwave becomes challenging when you can't lift your arms.

Sweating to the Oldies

Of the friends I interviewed about their fitness routines, the ones who had a consistent and healthy relationship with exercise—even if that meant subscribing to the cult of SLT or SoulCycle—all reported that it detoxed their minds just as much as it did their bodies.

This is a concept that Michelle Segar explores in her book *No Sweat: How the Simple Science of Motivation Can Bring You a Lifetime of Fitness*. Segar's research has shown that if your exercise attitude is solely based on numerical results—even the goals set by your fitness tracker—you won't stick with a long-term exercise routine. And more generic rewards like "good health" and "weight loss" don't motivate people enough on their own to sustain better behavior either. They're too abstract. Rather, it's the immediate emotional rewards that have the biggest impact.

The key was to approach physical activity from the vantage point of nourishment and energy rather than bodily control or guilt.

My motivations for my month of movement were much more in line with the self-care side of things than any sense of shame (though I felt plenty of it on my Megaformer). But I did realize that in struggling to keep up I had lost sight of the immediate mental reward that exercise could bring.

I needed to refind the fun.

As I thought about how our exercise culture has morphed from the camaraderie of organized sports to the shame-filled world of *The Biggest Loser*, I couldn't help but wonder what one of the forefathers of group fitness would make of all of this.

Before he became the proud owner of a closet full of bedazzled leotards and a fitness dynasty with equal panache, Richard Simmons was just another overweight teen in the South struggling to take control of his body. After years of fad dieting and over-the-counter pills, Simmons finally lost the excess weight by finding balance in food and movement. And with his own unique brand of crazy and genuine empathy for the physically challenged, he started his Beverly Hills studio, Slimmons.

When I went to the studio's website, it seemed to be just as stuck in the oldies as Richard's favorite playlists. But there was something refreshing about a fitness class model that had maintained its identity in the age of online sign-ups and forty-dollar fees. To see how people used to sweat it out at home, I ordered one of his first DVDs.

It had been a decade since I had last broken out my Tae Bo VHS tape, so it felt a little ridiculous putting on a sports bra and leggings just to groove by myself in the living room. After the first ten minutes of *Sweatin' to the Oldies*, I did begin to feel nostalgic for the energy of a live studio packed with people. But the joy 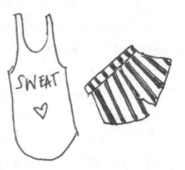 and acceptance that oozed out of Richard as he encouraged people of all shapes and sizes to get moving sprang straight from the screen and into my soul. It reminded me that you don't need to live in a big city with endless options in your backyard to find a trainer and a tune to groove to. And for me, part of that tune was laughter.

A month of playing in the trendy fitness sandbox caused me to forget about the types of movement I enjoyed most when I was growing up, the ones that left me breathless both from activity and from sheer joy: tennis matches, long hikes, casual bike rides, and afternoons cartwheeling in the grass. Bouncing on a trampoline had briefly brought back some of those sensations, but the intensity of the routine kept me from fully enjoying the high.

Alone in my apartment, I gained the freedom to be my own fitness flower. There was no judgment from anyone if I couldn't bounce or bend with the beat, and no instructor to shimmy me away from a much-needed water break. And without that added pressure, I found a kinder way to laugh at myself and actually enjoy my workout. That afternoon, I had a genuine smile on my face for the first time in my weeks of exercise. I may have felt like a fool, but I was a happy one, who had reconnected to the kind of movement that made her feel joyful and strong.

The Sweet Spot

Physical weakness was not the only thing that had caused my exercise habit to die a slow death. The other factor was self-employment.

I had reckoned with bad work habits during the back challenge. But I hadn't considered how my job trumped my exercise needs. All those immediate gratification points—focus, energy, and the feeling of well-being—too often got brushed aside in favor of crossing more items off my to-do list.

My thirty minutes of movement experiment helped shift my mindset on that front. It made me work walking breaks into my day in the same way I would have set aside time for lunch. And those walks ended up being more productive than I had ever given them credit for. In fact, one of my favorite parts was that it got me outside.

The extra vitamin D seemed like a worthwhile exchange for the endorphins I missed by not sprinting on a stationary bike for an hour. Plus, a quick walk around the block was easier to fit into my schedule and left me feeling less guilty than when I scooted away from my desk for an hour of aerobic twerking in a hot, crowded room.

On the other hand, while a gentle walk helped with productivity and creativity, I did see how more intense physical exercise could give my head a different type of release. Walking sometimes gave me too much leeway to brood; it twisted my mind like a windup toy instead of wearing it down. The total concentration required in a group fitness class was a distraction from all the negative emotions I had been fixated on. When I was bouncing ten feet in the air, I didn't have time to focus on any uncertainty in my professional or romantic future. The only self-doubt there was room for was worrying about flying through the air into the person next to me. And even that had to be pushed out of my mind so I could concentrate on what my limbs were doing in the moment.

These routines had the benefit of exhausting me upstairs and down. But the level of physical exhaustion didn't always feel therapeutic.

After trying out eight different studios, in the end I still preferred an hour of focused Pilates movements, relaxed vinyasas, and walk-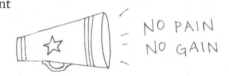ing outside over jumping, jiving, and spinning to deafeningly loud music. Yoga and Pilates teach you to respect your body and work around its limitations. Modifications aren't seen as a cop-out. Instead, they're necessary to improve your alignment and posture. And I felt a lot more supported in practices that emphasized that the quality of the journey was so much more powerful than the end result.

One of the few bright spots in my boutique fitness search was barre3, a barre-based class that was intense but lacked much of the machismo that dominated so many of the other exercises I tried. I ended up leaving feeling stronger, looser, and less sore than when I came, thanks to its philosophy of moderation and kindness. I wished that more instructors had promoted the idea of creating your own experience rather than pushing yourself to a point of being uncomfortable or destructive. To break through those internal walls like I was told to in "The Class," you shouldn't have to break down your body in the process.

I witnessed a few enthusiastic members of these fitness communities whose class frequency and drive put them in the addict or abuser camp yet never got told to slow down or give their bodies a rest. Instead, they were glorified.

When I decided to finally pop my spin cherry, I chose to ease into it at a slightly less cultish studio with brighter lights and more clientele over thirty. Halfway into the ride, after a long hill to the chorus of Miley Cyrus's "The Climb," the instructor got on the mic and announced that it was one of her regular student's four-hundredth ride of the year.

It was July.

The whole class erupted in cheerleader whoops and applause. Meanwhile, my jaw dropped. *Are you crazy?* I thought. That poor girl might have a problem. I'm not going to clap for that.

Despite not finding a high-intensity class that was a perfect fit, I had to admit that trying so many new movements left my body feeling very tight and nimble once I'd recovered from the soreness. All 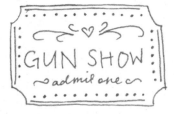 the physical insecurity I had felt around my back seemed to have gotten squeezed out during one rep of leg lifts or another. I noticed that long days logged in the kitchen didn't exhaust me in the same way they used to. I felt strong again. And with that outer strength came a different type of inner confidence. After years of blaming my body for my weakness, it was great to see what we could do once we started working together as a team again. I might have already found my happy medium—an exercise routine that distracted my mind without overly taxing my muscles—in one yoga or Pilates class a week, and taking a breather outside every day, but I was grateful that these fitness experiments helped me relocate my power.

Master health guinea pig Tim Ferriss said it best: the fastest way to change your inner game is to change your outer game. I hadn't exactly abided by the slow and gentle return to fitness that my autoimmune disease dictated, but by facing my physical fears, I'd successfully jumped many mental hurdles that, in Dr. John Sarno's eyes, might just lead to less future injury. If I could survive Megaformers, trampolines, dance routines, and lady Viking battle cries, I was pretty sure my mind and body were ready for anything.

As is the case with all wellness choices, exercise is extremely personal. Some of the things that didn't feed my fitness soul might feed yours. Here are some ways to reframe and maximize your experience with exercise, no matter what type of movement you enjoy most.

1. *If you can't afford a fancy fitness tracker, buy a pedometer.* You don't really know where you stand until you start monitoring your real-time numbers. In the long term, I'd rather just internalize what a good movement day feels like than rely on a report. But if you want some accountability in the beginning for a fraction of the price, buy an old-school pedometer (fifteen dollars). It may not look as cool as a fancy wristband or sync with an app, but the data is much more accurate. Wear it for a week to get a baseline calculation and then modify your routines from there.

2. *Make your city or surroundings into your outdoor gym.* One of A. J. Jacobs's biggest learnings in his book *Drop Dead Healthy* was the concept of "Guerilla Exercise." In order to squeeze physical activity into every spare minute of the day, Jacobs started to literally run errands, do wall push-ups in the bathroom stall, and opt for stairs instead of the elevator.

3. *Find something that feeds your mind as much as your body.* The sweet spot for exercise is finding that balance between the mental and physical. Some people like to drown out their worries with loud music and adrenaline. Others, like me, prefer to get quiet with themselves on a walk or in a yoga class. Finding that

middle ground can be huge for your mind and spirit, as well as your midsection.

4. *Don't be afraid to modify movements.* "Replace the 'no pain, no gain' mantra with 'work smarter, not harder' when exercising," said barre3 founder Sadie Lincoln in her response to the One Big Question. "One simple and highly effective way to do this is to modify postures so you feel really good while you're working out and even better afterward." In group scenarios, there's no shame in resting in child's pose, taking a water break, or deviating from the group's routine if a teacher gives you an easier option.

5. *Put exercise on your calendar like you would a meeting or doctor's appointment.* Prepaying for classes helps you commit to actually going. If you're exercising on your own time, though, scheduling is a powerful tactic to make sure you don't keep pushing it off.

6. *Try a class more than once.* The better you know the routines, the more comfortable you will be doing them and the more fun you'll have. Oftentimes you can get two-for-one beginner packages. I recognize that in most classes, my baseline for enjoyment might have improved once I knew what to expect.

7. *Get to know a teacher; drink the Kool-Aid if you have to.* There's a reason certain classes sell out so fast, and it's usually the teacher. Besides expertise, forming a relationship with your fearless leader means he or she will be up to date on your injuries and goals and better able to help you find success over time.

8. *Invest in the wardrobe.* I'm never going to be the person who buys a fierce cheetah-print sports bra to match her cheetah-print leggings. But looking the part *does* do something for your

commitment. Fashion can be a way to get excited about exercise—
Richard Simmons certainly knew that!

9. *Don't let calories burned justify unhealthy eating choices.* Eating smarter has a more profound effect on weight loss than exercising more. You don't want good exercise habits to undo your
progress on the balanced eating front. If you tend to be starving
before workouts, make a batch of my Green Egg (No Ham) Frittata Bites (page 218), or enjoy a little Thai Peanut Hummus with
Farmer's Market Crudités (page 220) for a quick fix afterward.

10. *Get enough rest.* In addition to taking breaks from exercise, getting adequate sleep is just as important when it comes to fueling
recovery, avoiding injury, and maximizing weight loss. Hence, why
improving my time under the sheets was next on my wellness
to-do list.

GREEN EGG (NO HAM) FRITTATA BITES

Makes 12 bites

If you like to get your workout over with in the morning but don't want to exercise on an empty stomach, these make-ahead frittata bites are a great grab-'n'-go breakfast and pre-workout snack. Eating a high-protein meal in the morning will leave you fuller for longer, and much less likely to have an energy crash, which is especially important before hitting the pavement.

....

2 tablespoons olive oil, plus more for greasing

2 small shallots, thinly sliced

5 ounces baby spinach or arugula, coarsely chopped

$1/4$ cup finely chopped sun-dried tomatoes (about 6)

$1/2$ teaspoon sea salt

8 large eggs

$1/2$ cup unsweetened almond or organic whole milk

1 ounce ($1/4$ cup) finely grated aged manchego or pecorino cheese

$1/4$ teaspoon freshly ground black pepper

1. Preheat the oven to 350°F.

2. In a large skillet, heat the olive oil over medium-high heat. Add the shallots and sauté until soft and beginning to brown, about 5 minutes. Add the spinach and cook until wilted, about 3 minutes. Remove the skillet from the heat, stir in the sun-dried tomatoes, and season lightly with salt. Set aside to cool slightly.

3. Meanwhile, in a 4-cup liquid measuring cup with a spout, whisk the eggs and milk until the whites are completely incorporated. Add the cheese, ½ teaspoon salt, and black pepper.

4. Grease or spray a muffin pan with olive oil. Divide the egg mixture between the prepared cups and add a rounded tablespoon of the greens mixture to each, making sure there's ¼ inch of room left. (They will puff up!)

5. Bake for 20 minutes, or until the frittata bites are golden brown around the edges. Let them cool in the pan until they pull away from the sides, about 5 minutes. Slide a silicone spatula around the edges to loosen the frittatas. Unmold and serve warm—the bites can be stored in the fridge for up to 4 days and reheated.

HEALTHY HEDONIST TIPS

While I tried not to eat dairy during my anti-inflammatory challenge (and still strive to limit it), eggs and cheese are a marriage made in healthy hedonist heaven. Goat and sheep's milk tend to have less lactose, meaning they're easier to digest than cow's milk. Aging also reduces the lactose content, so when I'm going for broke at the cheese counter, I try to stick to a hard, sharp pecorino or manchego. For soft cheeses, opt for goat cheese or a Greek feta, which is usually made with a mixture of cow and goat's milk.

MARKET SWAPS

If you've got a bunch of greens in your fridge (arugula, chard, kale), sub their chopped leaves for the spinach. This recipe is also a great place to use up any wayward wilting herbs. Simply use a cup of chopped herbs for the sautéed greens and add them to the egg mixture raw.

THAI PEANUT HUMMUS WITH FARMER'S MARKET CRUDITÉS

Serves 4 to 6

There are some store-bought condiments that aren't worth your time to DIY. But hummus couldn't be easier to make, and it's a great dish to add to your batch-cooking repertoire if you're a big snacker (especially post-workout). This version uses peanut butter instead of the usual Mediterranean tahini paste, along with lime juice and fresh mint leaves for a Thai spin. Prep the crudités and store them in individual containers so you always have carrot sticks and dip at the ready.

....

One 15-ounce can chickpeas (or 2 cups cooked), rinsed and drained

$^1/_4$ cup organic unsalted peanut butter

2 small garlic cloves

Zest of 1 lime

$^1/_4$ cup freshly squeezed lime juice (from about 2 limes)

$^1/_4$ cup (loosely packed) fresh mint leaves

$^1/_2$ teaspoon sea salt

$^1/_4$ teaspoon cayenne pepper

1 tablespoon finely chopped peanuts, for garnish

1 bunch of baby carrots (or 2 medium), trimmed and halved lengthwise

1 bunch of radishes, trimmed and quartered

1 small English cucumber, cut into sticks

1. In the bowl of a small food processor or blender, combine the chickpeas, peanut butter, garlic, lime zest, lime juice, mint leaves, ¼ cup water,

salt, and cayenne pepper. Puree, adding more water 1 tablespoon at a time if necessary, until the mixture is very smooth.

2. Transfer to a serving bowl and garnish with the chopped peanuts. Arrange the carrots, radishes, and cucumbers around the bowl and serve, or store the hummus for up to 2 weeks in the fridge.

HEALTHY HEDONIST TIPS

Peanuts are a high pesticide crop, so I recommend investing in organic. If you're allergic, you can always swap tahini or almond butter, but you won't get as much of a play on Thai peanut sauce.

MARKET SWAPS

You can sub cilantro or scallions for the mint. Use whatever produce is in season as your dippers. Broccoli, cauliflower, zucchini, green beans—they all make for delicious crudités. But if serving to company, I love how radishes make the plate look like you're at a fancy French party (even if you're serving Thai–Middle Eastern fusion).

PILLOW TALK

HITTING THE SNOOZE BUTTON

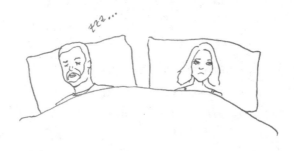

*On embracing the sanctity of sleep and turning bedtime
into the most productive part of my day.*

My bed and I have historically had a tortured relationship. As a hyperactive child, I had so much trouble winding down at the end of the day that my parents often resorted to a cocktail of melatonin, valerian root drops, and catnip (which has the opposite effect on humans than it does on felines) to get me to sleep. My mind was usually the culprit. In college, it would sometimes race so much thinking about exams and jobs and boys that I stayed up until morning in a state of to-do list mental mania.

Back then, I was young enough to muscle through the repercussions of sleepless nights, and they soon became a central part of my work ethic; with the help of Diet Coke from the library vending machine and my roommate's Ritalin, I regularly pulled "All-Night Tuesdays" to get all my papers out of the way and leave the rest of the week for the most important part of my education, partying.

Of course, that all changed after my Hashimoto's diagnosis.

Having embraced being a low-grade insomniac for most of my life, my body's new unquenchable need for sleep and my inability to function without it was one of the autoimmune symptoms I had the hardest time coming to terms with. I felt guilty when I didn't prioritize rest, and I often felt guiltier when I missed a night out with friends in order to log more of it. Since the vice detox, though, I had started to understand exactly how a bad night's sleep affected my waking hours. When I stayed up past my eleven p.m. bedtime, even if I'd only had one glass of wine, I would be operating with my head underwater the next day.

My next challenge: getting the doctor-recommended eight hours of sleep every night. Though needs vary among individuals, most researchers and medical professionals agree that anything less than six hours is definitely not enough. Only a small portion of the population (5 percent) is genetically predisposed to function on fewer.

My standard rationalization for All-Night Tuesday was that sleep is cumulative. Like my friend Sarah's father always told her growing up, you can take money out of your sleep piggy bank, but eventually you'll have to redeposit what you've borrowed. Medical professionals agree with this analogy in the short term so long as you make up for those lost z's within a few days. But if you're a night owl like I was in college, it's very unlikely you're going to be able to account for a ten-hour deficit over the weekend.

Our collective sleep debt has been slowly rising over the last century. Americans currently average 6.8 hours a night, down more than an hour since 1942, and two since the turn of the twentieth century. Between juggling the pressures of work, a busy social life, and the need to spend quality time with those closest to us, sleep is often the priority that gets compromised first. To complete all of our obligations and still stay up to date on who will die on the latest episode of *Game of Thrones*, many of us adopt Ben Franklin's MO: we can sleep when we're dead.

And yet studies have shown that sleep deprivation can reduce your life span by raising blood pressure and, by extension, increasing risk of stroke and heart attack. It also taxes the immune system, which can be especially difficult for those of us dealing with autoimmune and adrenal issues. Being unconscious under the sheets sets the stage for many of our body's essential biological functions: growth, memory storage, detoxification, immunity, and energy regeneration. A few recent studies have even linked subpar sleep to an increased risk of Alzheimer's. The list is enough to keep a troubled sleeper like me up at night.

Despite my body's cravings, committing to going to bed on time wasn't enough. Exercise month had helped me fall asleep more easily once I hit the pillow, but I still often found myself tossing and turning in the night, my shirt damp with sweat, my mind fixated on how every missed moment would affect my morning. I wanted to figure out what was dooming my bedtime hours to be the waste of time I'd always feared. Was one measly late-night cocktail really disrupting my most beneficial sleep stages, as research suggested it did? Or might there be other factors, like the person making the deafening sounds of a dying piglet next to me? Some of these issues might be easier to fix than others, but regardless, I wanted to live the hours I spent awake in ways that would set me up for success under the sheets.

Pressing the Snooze Button

I'd actually been wrestling with this challenge for several months before I took it in earnest. At the writers' colony in Tennessee, I decided to do something crazy: I didn't set an alarm.

I had been talking with my friend Amie Valpone, a fellow cookbook author and natural foods chef, and was inspired to hear how aggressively dedicated she was to following her body's circadian rhythm. In her book, *Eating Clean: The 21-Day Plan to Detox, Fight Inflammation, and Reset Your Body*, Amie shares how eliminating the foods and products that taxed her fragile system helped her overcome ten years of chronic illness. But she also confided in me that there's even more to detoxing your life than what you put in or on your body; you also have to let yourself rest. Amie's trick for getting enough sleep was not to schedule any meetings or calls until noon so she could let her body dictate her wake-up time. Some nights she needed ten to twelve hours to reboot, others less. She thoroughly believed that any time spent healing herself was worthwhile, no matter how long it took. And what could require less effort on that front than sleeping?

This strategy clearly wouldn't be feasible for anyone tethered to the Man's early bird schedule. Even as a freelancer, the idea of starting my workday at lunchtime sounded aspirational but potentially anxiety-producing. I could justify a mid-afternoon yoga class every now and then, but the culturally accepted convention of "you snooze, you lose" weighed too heavily on my workaholic soul to risk being unconscious until noon on a Monday, lest I need to log an All-Night Tuesday to make up for it.

Going alarm-free in the counter-reality of an isolated cabin in the woods in some ways may have been a cop-out, but for a control freak like myself, it was a safe way to check in with my circadian rhythm and see whether, in a quiet, dark, Charlie-free sleep utopia, it still existed.

THE FIRST FEW DAYS of my writers' retreat, letting my body be my guide worked surprisingly well. Exhausted from travel, I passed out at eleven p.m. and woke up with the sunrise at seven. But by the third night, the cynic in my subconscious emerged.

Being alone in the middle of the
woods was less of a Thoreauvian
fantasy than a modern-day nightmare
in the making. A particularly vivid
dream about being sold into sex slavery
starring the cast of *Winter's Bone* left
me wide-awake in a clammy funk for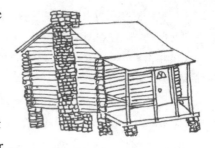
hours. I fell back asleep just before sunrise and, without an alarm, my
body didn't stir again until after lunchtime. When my eyes finally fluttered open and saw the clock, I was seized by a productivity panic.

The following nights were equally restless. At the end of my stay,
I felt relaxed from being away from the city and nourished from all
the homemade meals I'd cooked for myself, but I didn't feel completely recharged and renewed. Instead, after two weeks of going to bed
early and sleeping in, I'd found myself back in a vicious cycle of
insomnia.

Watching the Clock

Only a small percentage of people suffer from the true definition of
insomnia, which is total sleeplessness. More colloquially, the term can
be applied to anyone who has issues falling asleep or experiences frequent periods of wakefulness during the night—roughly a third of the
population.

On paper, these poor sleepers suffer from an efficiency issue. You can
measure this by looking at the ratio of how much time you spend in bed
compared to how much of that time you actually spend sleeping. In Tennessee, my efficiency rate was so low, I'm pretty sure I wouldn't have even
qualified to work next to Lucille Ball at a candy factory.

Back home when I ran into this issue many nights in a row, I didn't reach for a combination of melatonin, valerian root drops, and catnip. Instead, I resorted to the adult equivalent of my parents' sleep potion: Ambien.

Despite his best efforts to get me to bed as a child, my dad has been a big role model for high-functioning insomnia. I've never known him to sleep through the night, which was unfortunate in high school, when I'd attempt to sneak in after curfew only to find a shadowy figure in the front hallway eating oatmeal in his boxers. Seeing how reliant my father was on pills and yet how infrequently they actually worked helped temper my use of medication to only emergency situations: when I was overly anxious or already owed my sleep creditors a big chunk of change. But as part of finding a better path forward on the sleep front, I wanted to put my Ambien prescription to bed for good.

The problem with sleeping pills, besides the late-night carbs, is that with physical dependency comes tolerance. And the more you have to take, the more your morning-after droopiness can rival the aftermath of an All-Night Tuesday.

Because hypnotic medications reduce the deepest, most important portions of your sleep cycle, they don't always leave your body or mind feeling well rested. Studies have even shown that sleeping pill usage leads to impaired memory function by reducing the time spent in the brain's restorative REM (rapid eye movement) phase. More important, pills don't do anything to fix the underlying behavior that's causing your sleepless-ness in the first place.

As I wandered the Internet in search of an app or program that would improve my sleep efficiency, I was surprised to find that in many clinical trials, cognitive behavioral therapy (or CBT)—a goal-oriented type of treatment that changes the patterns of thinking that are behind people's problems—outperformed sleeping pills in fighting insomnia.

I immediately purchased an e-course specifically for sleep issues with a simple five-week PDF protocol. As I read through the techniques,

I learned why my alarm clock moratorium in Tennessee had been so misguided.

It turns out that routine is the most important tactic for building better bedtime habits. You can train yourself onto any sleep cycle so long as your body knows what's coming and can adapt. I had missed this by diving into a new sleep system with another person's best practices and not enough research on what would work best for my particular set of problems.

The manual explained that sleeping in on weekends is one of the reasons why Sunday night insomnia is so common. Although you might think it's just your Monday morning worries meddling with your mind, the inability to fall asleep is often due to a lack of "prior wakefulness." The longer you can go between rising and going back to bed, the more likely you'll be to pass out.

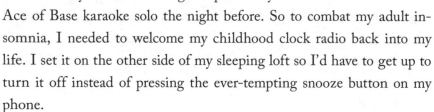

To give your body the routine it craves, the first rule of CBT for insomnia is to stick to a firm wake-up time, even on weekends, regardless of how late you took the stage to perform your Ace of Base karaoke solo the night before. So to combat my adult insomnia, I needed to welcome my childhood clock radio back into my life. I set it on the other side of my sleeping loft so I'd have to get up to turn it off instead of pressing the ever-tempting snooze button on my phone.

JUST AS SLEEPING IN isn't always the solution for a better night's sleep, neither is getting into bed early. In fact, it can actually make insomnia worse.

As C. S. Lewis once said, "many things—such as loving, going to sleep, or behaving unaffectedly—are done worst when we try hardest to do them." In Tennessee, the stress of pursuit turned my bed into a cue for wide-awake frustration instead of serene rest.

Rather than forcing myself into bed when I wasn't tired, I used the CBT instructions to calculate what my *earliest* possible bedtime should be based on how many hours I usually slept. Trying to go from six hours a night to eight is just as difficult as jumping straight from running a half marathon to the full twenty-six miles. You have to slowly condition your body to sleep more to avoid the mental hula-hooping that results when you put too much pressure on yourself.

In order to optimize these scheduling adjustments, though, I also needed to address my sleep hygiene.

Bedroom Bad Behavior

When I first moved into my small studio in Manhattan, I thought I had won the rental lottery. The neighborhood was just hitting its Yuppie stride, and somehow I had managed to find a reasonably affordable, recently renovated condo.

As anyone who's ever tried to score an apartment in New York City knows, you usually have to show up with your checkbook in hand and, if the property looks remotely promising, be ready to sign away your life's savings on the spot to secure it. Because of this accelerated timeline, it's common for potential annoyances to go unnoticed or get downplayed as atmospheric quirks. When I saw the high ceilings, the Edison light fixtures, and the full-size fridge, it was easy to overlook the fact that the apartment was located directly above a sports bar and a Mexican restaurant more popular for its four-dollar margarita drink special than its authentic mole sauce. Instead of considering whether or not I wanted to sleep in a crawl space with a ceiling four feet above my head for the next few years, I went home and immediately wrote the landlords a love letter to make my check stand out from the five other applicants in line ahead of me.

Now, as I lay wide-awake listening to the smokers having a lover's quarrel outside my window, I cursed my powers of persuasion. Having a dark, quiet, chilly room—one of the best ways to ensure good "sleep hygiene"—was apparently the price I had to pay for big windows and a dishwasher.

My crawl space did have its advantages. There wasn't a whole lot you could do up there besides read, so that helped fulfill the requirement of reserving the bedroom just for sleep and sex. It was stark and streamlined. There were no piles of clothing strewn across the bed, no glowing electronic appliances, no wall art or pictures that were outside the sleep-friendly color palette of light soothing blues.

But without spending thousands of dollars on blackout curtains or uglifying my apartment with cheap paper ones, I was never going to be able to block out the neon green glow of the LED tequila worm sign hanging outside my window. A warm room makes it harder for your body temperature to drop to a sleep-ready setting. And because heat rises, my sleeping loft made overcoming this issue extra difficult. Earplugs and a strong fan helped combat the noise and cool me down, but I was never going to get the type of peace and quiet of a log cabin in the woods— especially not with the added barnyard din of Charlie's snoring on nights he slept over.

Since there was little more I could do to make my environment have stronger sleep cues, I decided to focus my energy on the hygiene violations I was accruing outside the bedroom.

Bright Lights, Big City

Many modern comforts contribute to our bodies not being fully ready for rest by bedtime. A mid-afternoon coffee break means caffeine is still in your system at night; late dinners force your body to work on digesting food when it should be engaging in less energetic activities; and binge-watching a crime drama leaves you filled with adrenaline instead of relaxed and ready for dreamland.

The latter falls under the category of stimulus control. It's best to avoid anything that's going to agitate your mind before bed, be it an annoying email from your boss or a plot twist that you'll be pulling apart for hours. But even if you're zoning out to a Bob Ross waterscape, many electronics we use have the added issue of blue light.

The invention of round-the-clock light sources has had the biggest impact on our circadian rhythms of any modern convenience. The blue light emitted by the sun is now also mimicked by our television, computer, tablet, phone, and, for some of us, a neon LED tequila worm. This inhibits our natural production of melatonin, the main hormone that programs our internal clocks for sleep.

Normally, our melatonin levels start increasing after sundown and lower with the first light of morning. But when we come home after dark and hop on an electronic device, our bodies get very different sleep memos. One study found that our systems are so sensitive, even blind people can have their circadian rhythms thrown off by exposure to blue light.

Since I didn't think I could realistically get all my stimuli under control before sundown, I devised an alternate set of strategies to keep my internal clock in sync with the outside world.

There are a few apps these days that can help block blue light on your devices. I downloaded f.lux on my computer to sync the screen color with the time of day; for other pre-bed electronic activities, I ordered a pair of orange glasses. The only options available on Amazon looked like something Dick Cheney would wear to the gun range. But one Swiss study measured the effect of these blue light–blocking shades on a group of teenage boys and found that 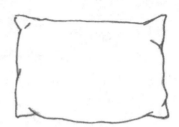 they felt significantly more tired at bedtime when they wore them. So I gave it a whirl. TV isn't free of blue light, but because of the distance to your face, phones and tablets are worse. Before my glasses arrived, when I could, I tried reading on Charlie's Kindle, which doesn't emit the same type of light. It was also a good excuse to pick up some bound paper from the stacks of cookbooks and food magazines I was no longer using as a makeshift laptop stand.

Finally, there was more work to be done in the morning.

Keeping my alarm clock set for a consistent time and kicking my snooze button habit had already been helpful. Even if I'd had a sub-par sleep and was too tired to get up, it meant my sleep was that much sounder the subsequent night, thanks to the power of "prior wakeful-ness." One solution for waking up more easily and keeping my hormones in sync was to simply step outside. Sunlight causes your skin to produce vitamin D naturally, and vitamin D is melatonin's counterpart. A walk around the block or exposure to a bright window first thing in the morning stops melatonin production and rewires your internal tempera-ture cycle to rise earlier in the a.m., and consequently dip earlier in the evening.

I hoped that these strategies would at least take care of my first effi-ciency issue: drifting off quickly and easily. The thing that remained a bigger mystery was how to wrangle my mind to then stay asleep.

Dream a Little Dream of Me

Charlie was becoming increasingly aware of his role in my sleeplessness.

During the honeymoon phase of our relationship, exhaustion seemed like a worthy trade-off for two young, busy professionals trying to get to know each other better, usually late at night, after various commitments ended and we could converge in the same bedroom. But after a few months, I became more and more grumpy about the fact that my night-owl boyfriend was keeping me up past my bedtime, and then ensuring I got even less sleep once under the sheets, thanks to his nasal orchestra of wheezes, grunts, and snorts.

So for our one-year anniversary, in lieu of jewelry or concert tickets, Charlie gave me what I wanted most: the gift of sleep.

I was beaming with excitement when I unwrapped the fancy new sleep monitor for my bedside table. It wouldn't necessarily fix my nightly soundtrack so much as drown it out with an array of ocean waves hitting the shoreline. But the device had other enticing functions—mainly as an objective party to transcribe my sleep diary.

Two weeks of using the CBT handwritten log had left me unsure of my own accuracy. Without watch-ing the clock (which was forbidden), it was impossi-ble to know exactly how long Charlie's snoring had kept me lying awake. My new device detected the movement of my upper body while I slept. Not only would it log a more precise quantity, but it could also tell me how I was doing on quality.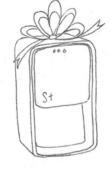

One thing that we can't possibly measure ourselves is how much time we spend in the most necessary, restorative parts of our sleep cycle.

Our nights begin with light sleep, where you're so easily awoken that most people don't even think they're sleeping at all. Next, you delve into a deeper sleep, when the brain activity slows down. Being woken up during this stage can leave you disoriented and unable to perform complex actions like driving or brushing your teeth without getting toothpaste spittle all over the mirror. The final stage is REM sleep, which makes up 20 percent of our cycle and gets its name from the eye-rolling taking place during it. If you were to lift your lids, it would look like your dreams were a highlight reel of parental nagging and corny jokes.

While you dream in other stages, REM is when the majority of them occur, a mysterious by-product of all the cognitive shop-keeping taking place. Other than the movement happening behind your eyelids, every muscle is completely paralyzed. This can be thought of as a biological safeguard against acting out any particularly vivid activities. (The dramatic game of dream soccer that left me with three broken toes in high school must have taken place during a different stage.)

The sleep machine came in very handy for tracking how much time I was actually spending in deep and REM sleep. On nights of extreme restlessness, when my mind was suicide bombing itself, the time I spent tossing and turning was often not as long as it felt in the moment. It was reassuring to know how much of my morning-after assessments had been amplified by self-pity. And knowing that I hadn't failed as badly as I thought made me more positive about the subsequent night's sleep.

Of course, this also went the other way. Even if I'd gone to bed for an eight-hour time slot (which was hard enough in the first place), the bio-motion sleep sensor might give me a C+ thanks to not enough time spent in the REM stage. This would make me feel down-and-out the next day, and only partially from exhaustion. It ignited my perfectionism, shaming my subconscious for not doing a good enough job overnight.

The machine also confirmed that when it came to sleeping soundly throughout the night, Charlie was, indeed, part of my problem, which was probably not what he wanted from an object meant to commemorate our year of love.

Two Very Different Spoons

Sleeping as a pair has largely escaped scientific analysis. Most medical studies are confined to labs where the behavior of one person is monitored. And yet in the real world, a shared bed is the cultural norm. How can you adequately evaluate someone's sleep patterns in a clinical setting without a partner snorting, flailing, and teeth grinding a few inches away?

"For women, sleep is a sensual and emotional experience, embedded in a complex system in which the environment plays an important role," Gerhard Klösch writes in his book *Sleeping Better Together.* Men, on the other hand, don't ascribe so much meaning to it; sleep is a biological need, and any other details are of little interest. "The result is that men are less bothered by a subpar sleeping space, and they can sleep well despite just about any atmospheric deficiencies."

That women suffer disproportionately from sleep disorders makes sense when you also consider that men are disproportionately the biggest snorers. If you can sleep through your own racket, isn't it much less likely that you'll be disturbed by anything else?

The longer a relationship lasts, the more personal sleeping habits begin to dominate. Now that the rainbows and butterflies were behind us, Charlie and I were right on schedule for a bedroom come-to-Jesus moment. Since there's really only so much you can do about incompatible schedules and blocked nasal passages, finding other compromises meant we would have to put all our sleep cards on the table, including an issue that could actually be removed: our third sleeping companion, the dog.

. . .

BARON THE BEAGLE had been Charlie's primary cuddle buddy, sleeping partner, and best friend for ten years. His entitlement to a place in the bed was so cemented that he'd even been given a custom-built wooden staircase to come and go as he pleased. When Charlie would pull up a third chair to the table so Baron could join us for a romantic meal, I wasn't thrilled, but when it came to the bedroom, his intrusions made me far more uncomfortable.

If the bed was supposed to be a sacred space reserved for sleep and sex, I can't begin to say what being in physical contact with a hairy beagle did for my enjoyment of both those acts. The old saying that no one can come between a man and his dog becomes ever truer when said dog has wedged himself under the covers as a physical divider.

"It's like having an ex-girlfriend sleeping with you, night after night," one friend commiserated. "If you don't feel like you're number one in bed, how can that not affect every other part of your relationship?"

A study conducted by the Mayo Clinic found that 53 percent of pet owners said their sleep was disrupted on a daily basis by their animals. Among the factors cited were nocturnal wanderings, dream-induced kicking, and loud snoring by dogs. I was suffering from all of the above.

Intimacy issues aside, Baron also doubled the noise violations.

Which is why when Charlie asked me over dinner if I wanted to move in together, my response was not one that either of us might have hoped for when discussing the next chapter of our future: as far as the bed was concerned, it was either the dog or me. The topic of sharing an apartment couldn't be on the table until I knew I wouldn't have to sacrifice my sleep in order to live in it.

Despite this ultimatum, Charlie dragged his feet for weeks. He removed the stairs, which did nothing to prevent Baron from lunging onto the bed (his sizable girth belied the fact that he was very nimble). And it turns out that having forty pounds landing hard on your tibia is worse than just being walked all over at three a.m. After a weeklong stalemate during which I retreated to my own apartment, Charlie finally lofted the bed.

It took a few nights with the dog a comfortable three feet below for me to realize Charlie's reluctance wasn't so much about the dog's needs, it was about his own. I had ripped away his security blanket. As his first real adult girlfriend, I was forcing him to set boundaries and make room. And though I felt guilty about causing this separation anxiety, banishing Baron was a gesture that I badly needed in order to feel supported in the bedroom and beyond.

The Sweet Spot

Once I had the sleep monitor, it was even easier to see how my choices during the day affected my night. I did indeed fall asleep quickly and easily when I'd gone to Pilates and eaten a light, early meal—and even more so when I slept solo.

It was harder to tell what my blue light strategies accomplished. There was not enough lingerie in the world to offset making orange glasses a consistent part of my nighttime wardrobe. Plus, I found that reading of any sort, even if done on a blue light device, helped me get in a better headspace for sleep. Falling asleep was the biggest problem when my mind was running in circles, and concentrating on someone else's words helped reel it in.

In general, the most useful part of the cognitive behavioral therapy program was liberating myself from the mental roadblocks I'd built around my sleep habits. Sticking to a consistent morning wake-up time and getting some sunshine in the morning helped me feel fatigued by night-fall, which was a better reminder to get home at a reasonable hour than looking at my watch and stressing about what would happen if I didn't.

If you feel anxious about an impending bad night's sleep—or label it as such before it's even happened due to a late bedtime—like those back attacks, it's very likely to be a self-fulfilling prophecy. The program's biggest gift was reminding me that going to bed past curfew wasn't the end of the world. And that made savoring the last hour of the day with Charlie feel like less of a handicap to my health.

Our pillow talk was a time for stream-of-consciousness confessions, trivial gossip, and downloading each other's daily narrative. And as with my most cherished middle school girlfriends, part of that sleepover high was always having one more thing to say after the light was turned off. Knowing that my sleep might not suffer from prolonging this intimate part of the day allowed me to relax and enjoy the precious time together instead of being paranoid about how his presence was affecting my beauty rest.

MORE SO THAN any other area of my wellness, my sleep experiments proved that despite my best-laid plans, there were only so many variables I could bend in my favor. Consistent wake-up and bedtimes were hard to maintain when they didn't mesh with those of the person next to me or were overshadowed by 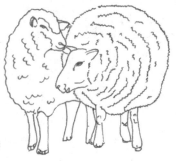 bigger problems. Sharing a bed made sleeping a team sport—we needed to confront the issues together.

I won't downplay how much more joy I felt getting into clean sheets and not having to stress about laying my sensitive skin on a pillow covered in dog hair, or worry about being awoken by a paw to the abdomen.

But in terms of my ability to sleep, just getting Baron out of the bed was not a perfect solution. Now there was the sound of his nails clack-clacking on the wood as he wandered in the night, and his clawing at the door in the morning to be let out before the alarm went off. And since he was farther away, it was also harder to rouse him from his doggy night terrors, which, for beagles, involve a lot of howling.

I knew that this was as far as I could push Charlie, though. So I had to try not to be so bitter about it. The more self-righteous I got in my head about the unfairness of my sleep situation, the more the insomnia devil on my shoulder grew, especially if those thoughts occurred at three a.m. to the soundtrack of Baron chasing rabbits in his dreams.

I knew I needed to try to remember all of the positive reasons for sleeping in the same room together, even as a threesome.

Deep in the thicket beyond the honeymoon phase, I still preferred sleeping with Charlie to sleeping without him. And I knew that in his willingness to dethrone his other bedtime companion, he felt the same way. After a few weeks, Charlie even admitted that he felt much more rested in the morning without the dog in the bed.

So though our sleep hygiene may have been a long way from fitting together like spoons, as long as our bodies did I decided I'd rather be side by side as 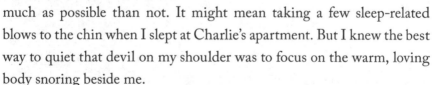 much as possible than not. It might mean taking a few sleep-related blows to the chin when I slept at Charlie's apartment. But I knew the best way to quiet that devil on my shoulder was to focus on the warm, loving body snoring beside me.

As we took the next step in sharing a life together, even more aspects of my wellness would become entwined with Charlie's. And the subject of my next set of challenges—fertility and the hormonal crapshoot known as contraception—was a conversation that would certainly need to be tackled with the help of my other half.

Healthy Hedonist Sleep Tips

Small sleep hygiene modifications do add up. But if you're unable to block out all of the noise and blue light from your night life, here are some other strategies for falling and staying asleep.

1. *Keep your alarm consistent.* Getting up at the same time every day helps give your body the routine it craves. Plus, the more "prior wakefulness" you've experienced, the easier it will be to fall asleep the subsequent night. If you suffer from insomnia, keep sleeping in to a minimum, even on weekends, so you don't throw off your cycle for the week ahead.

2. *Limit wakeful time in bed to half an hour.* That maximum time allotment goes for hanging out after hitting the snooze button in the morning as well as watching TV or reading before you nod off. You want your bed to have strong sleep cues. If you wake in the night and can't fall back asleep, get out of bed and only go back once you're feeling very drowsy. While you wait it out in another room, try reading a magazine instead of scrolling through your European friends' Instagram feeds so you're not wiring yourself further with blue light.

3. *Drink sleepy or tummy tea.* If your brain is keeping you up at night, try sipping something warm and soothing before bed. Acu Heidi believes that strengthening your digestion helps your body break down anything it takes in, be it food or information. Add grated fresh ginger, known to ease digestive issues, to your Sleepytime tea, or make the from-scratch version (page 245).

4. *Take a hot shower or bath.* A drop in body temperature is a key prelude to sleep. If your internal thermostat is off, one way to hack it is to take a ten-minute bath or shower. Though it's counterintuitive that a hot tub will cool your body temperature, the sharp rise brought on by the warm water will be followed by a sharp fall once you're out. Adding relaxing lavender bath salts and sipping ginger tea while in there is a sleep prep triple threat (in a good way).

5. *Don't eat or booze within two hours of bedtime.* As I discovered during detox month, your liver's main work shift is the middle of the night, from one to three a.m. It's important to let it concentrate on cleaning your blood instead of allocating energy to digestion. You might be tempted to use alcohol as a sleep aid, since it can help you fall into deep sleep quickly. But giving your liver this task can lead to disrupted REM sleep in the middle of the night.

6. *Keep a sleep diary.* Wristband trackers tend to be even more inaccurate for sleep than they are for movement. If you don't want to invest in a fancy tableside monitor like my S+ by ResMed, keep a journal to record your bedtime, wake-up time, how many disruptions you had in the night, and how long it took you to fall asleep. It might be hard to give exact times without looking at a clock, so just estimate. The CBT for Insomnia online program includes a helpful sleep diary worksheet.

7. *Use a mind-dump journal.* Writing down your anxieties before bed has a funny way of extracting them from your brain and tabling the mental conversation until morning.

8. *Give yourself a bedtime attitude adjustment.* Cognitive restructuring is a big part of CBT for insomnia. Instead of dwelling on how you'll suffer in the morning if you don't get enough sleep, remind yourself that you'll be fine. The more anxiety you have

about what the lack of sleep will do to you, the less likely you are to be able to wind down to a state where you can actually get some rest. As long as you have five hours of core sleep, you'll be able to function.

9. ***Check your phone at the bedroom door or turn it off.*** In the case of blue light, the length of exposure does matter. Ten minutes is much less jarring to your melatonin production than an hour. Try to keep your devices out of the bedroom or set them to airplane mode so you're not tempted to mindlessly browse the Internet before bed.

10. ***Manipulate your sleep senses with aromatherapy.*** Use scents to your advantage by adding lavender, vanilla, and jasmine essential oils, which have a calming effect, to your bedtime routine. You can put a few drops in your bath or rub a little on your chest. If your partner doesn't mind, you can even spray the bedroom or your pillow before getting under the sheets.

11. ***Choose a sacred night to refuel.*** I know that picking and choosing social plans so I can get eight hours of sleep will make me a better friend to others and myself. It's not just alcohol or sugar or gluten, but the hustle and bustle of a night on the town that overwhelms my sensitive system. Try to say yes to adventures that feed your spirit, not obligations that feel like drudgery. And a few nights a week—Sunday and Monday work well—clear your schedule to enjoy some downtime and add more coins to the sleep piggy bank.

DAD'S OVERNIGHT OATMEAL WITH ALMOND BUTTER AND DRIED CHERRIES

Serves 4 to 6

As I discovered on more than one occasion thanks to my father's insomniac eating sprees, there's no pot more annoying to clean than one that's been coated with sticky oatmeal and left to sit for hours. Whether you're eating it in the morning or as a midnight snack, overnight oatmeal is a delicious, no-cook solution. Simply stir all the ingredients together and then leave the mixture in the fridge for twelve hours, so the oats soften, the chia seeds plump, and the flavors come together. While this combination of whole grains and seeds is a great protein boost in the morning, I also discovered that my dad's usual dried cherries and almonds actually contain essential melatonin and tryptophan, which can prepare your body for the most productive type of late-night food coma.

....

1 cup unsweetened almond milk

$^1/_2$ cup mashed banana (from 2 medium bananas)

2 tablespoons almond butter

1 tablespoon maple syrup

$^1/_2$ teaspoon ground cinnamon

Pinch of sea salt

1 cup gluten-free old-fashioned rolled oats

$^1/_4$ cup unsweetened dried cherries

2 tablespoons chia seeds

1. In a medium bowl, stir together the almond milk, bananas, almond butter, maple syrup, cinnamon, and salt until smooth. Fold in the oats,

dried cherries, and chia seeds. Divide the oat mixture among individual ramekins, mason jars or bowls, or cover as is and refrigerate overnight.

2. Enjoy cold or reheated in the microwave for 30 seconds. For a gussied-up bowl, top with sliced banana, slivered almonds, and a dash of cinnamon. The overnight oats will keep for up to a week in the fridge.

HEALTHY HEDONIST TIPS

When you're buying dried fruit, make sure there's no added sugar. Cherries and cranberries in particular are often sweetened with apple or grape juice concentrate to make them less sour.

MARKET SWAPS

I've always thought peanut butter with banana was an even more dreamy combo than with jelly. Try subbing it for almond butter, using hemp milk instead of almond, and trading hemp seeds for chia. The end result will be an oatmeal version of one of my favorite smoothies: the banana hammock.

SLEEPY TUMMY TEA

Makes 2 cups

For packaged items that I consume every day, I've found it pays to make my own versions in bulk. Adapted from Emily Han, the amazing herbalist and author of Wild Drinks and Cocktails, *this Sleepy Tummy Tea recipe is one of the easiest to re-create. Spearmint and chamomile are two ingredients often found in store-bought nighttime formulas, and they have even more flavor when used whole instead of pre-ground in a tea bag. Fennel seeds and dried ginger are great for your digestion and can help soothe your stomach so it doesn't keep you up at night. This tea is wonderfully calming, with just a hint of menthol, anise, and spice in the background.*

....

1 teaspoon dried ginger root (see Market Swaps note), or 2 teaspoons
   minced fresh

1 teaspoon dried spearmint leaves

1 teaspoon fennel seeds

1 teaspoon dried chamomile flowers

2 cups boiling water

1. Place the ginger, spearmint, fennel seeds, and chamomile in a fine-mesh infuser. Pour the boiling water over the tea mix and allow to steep for 10 minutes.

2. Remove the infuser and enjoy.

HEALTHY HEDONIST TIPS

You can buy wholesale herbs online at www.MountainRoseHerbs.com. One 4-ounce bag of chamomile flowers is only eight dollars and will probably last the entire year. Make the Sleepy Tummy Tea mix in bulk and store in an airtight container for daily brewing. If you find yourself with an excess of chamomile flowers, they make a beautiful addition to a soothing, pre-bedtime bath!

MARKET SWAPS

To make your own dried ginger, peel and thinly slice a knob of ginger, then place it on a rimmed baking sheet. Leave it out on the counter for 1 to 2 days, mixing once, until the pieces are fully dry. The same technique works for lemon peel or zest, which would make a delicious addition. Try subbing lavender flowers for chamomile, or peppermint for spearmint.

RAG TIME

MOON SISTERHOOD AND THE STATE OF HORMONE HEALTH

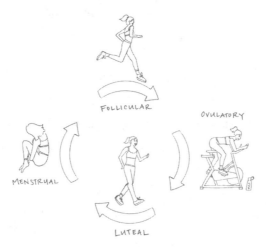

On periods, sex, and conscious contraception.

The biggest stepping-stone on my hormonal journey came six months prior to starting my project, as I made the reluctant decision to go off the pill.

When I first started taking it at sixteen, I wasn't having sex yet and was too immature to try to understand what was going on inside my body. Like the 58 percent of women who are on hormonal birth control for reasons other than contraception, my doctor gave it to me because my period was irregular. And I stayed on it for over a decade without a second thought.

Even after my autoimmune diagnosis, I operated under the misconception that my birth control pills were a necessary weight on the hormonal seesaw—that without them, my system couldn't maintain proper balance. My main gripe, the one that had gotten me hooked on synthetic hormones in the first place, was that the few times I had tried to go off,

I would get my period every two weeks. In high school that was torture. And though my black pants collection had expanded since then, it wasn't something I looked forward to experiencing again.

Eventually, though, thanks to another lecture by my militant Greek endocrinologist Dr. A, I had to come to terms with the fact that the strongest force regulating my hormones was also the very thing preventing me from fixing them for good.

As Dr. Christiane Northrup, the author of *Women's Bodies, Women's Wisdom*, writes, using birth control pills to regulate your period "is akin to putting a piece of tape over the flashing indicator light on the dashboard of your car and pretending you have addressed the engine problem, rather than looking under the hood and dealing with the underlying issue."

Despite the widespread, long-term use, there's been hardly any research on the effects of keeping your body on this synthetic cycle for so long—from fragile adolescence all the way through one's twenties. And many of the pill's opponents argue that its most devastating influence is that it brushes aside any alternate tactics for prevention of hormone-related disorders at an early age.

The endocrine system, of which the thyroid is a part, is a complex organizational chart of glands, each responsible for micromanaging specific hormones that control the body's various functions. Everything from our hair to our appetite to our mental clarity relies on the health of this ecosystem.

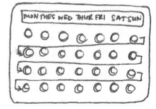

Today, over twenty million people have a thyroid-related disease, and women are five to eight times more likely to be at risk. At the same time, one in ten women suffer from endometriosis, and another five million endure polycystic ovary syndrome (PCOS). And whether or not it is a result of the rise of these endocrine-related diseases or other factors, one in ten couples have fertility issues.

In adolescence, the hormonal abnormalities for which the pill is being prescribed may not be so abnormal after all. It's a volatile time full of change, emotionally and physically. It can take up to four years of menstruating for a girl's body to adjust from child to woman and for her periods to become "regular." But instead of allowing for this to happen naturally, hormonal birth control changes the reproductive system—and our endocrine functions at large—before it has had a chance to fully develop.

You cannot take away a vital sign of a woman's reproductive health (ovulation) without playing with the hormonal motherboard as a child would a set of elevator buttons. The pill may be, in many ways, a pain reliever. But it's not a cure. True to my experience, those same symptoms for which it was prescribed can resurface the second you stop.

Miscontraceptions

When I went off the pill, right out of the gate, my outward appearance of wellness seemed to wash away with the precision and harshness of a Noxzema cleansing cloth. My scalp became itchy, oily, and flaky. My breasts shriveled back to the California raisins they had been in ninth grade. And my skin began to descend into the chaos that had sent me back through the revolving door of my dermatologist's office.

Dr. A said it could take six months to a year for my body to normalize. As the withdrawal dragged on, though, I worried that greasy scalp, inflamed skin, and unpredictable tummy troubles were my new normal. I desperately wanted to throw in the towel and reach for those plastic punch cards at the back of my medicine cabinet.

Ultimately, though, I came out the other side with a new clarity. When I stopped Yasmin, I finally started Nature-Throid, a hormone replacement medication to treat my Hashimoto's. Whether it was that butterfly-shaped gland coming back to life or my sex hormones or both, after a month my hot flashes and mental fog started to lift. And what I saw was that all of these symptoms weren't being caused by the absence of the pill; they had been lying in wait all along.

Why did I tape over the dashboard for so many years?

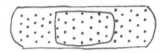

It took me until this project to understand that so many of my ongoing symptoms—insomnia, acne, headaches, digestive issues—were hormonally based. During my earlier wellness experiments, I'd covered some very necessary steps toward detoxing my life of endocrine disruptors—chlorine in drinking water, phthalates in beauty products, pesticides on vegetables, and artificial hormones from factory-farmed meat, just to name a few.

Controlling my blood sugar, which I did by cutting down on sweets and simple carbs, was also incredibly important for maintaining overall hormonal balance. As I learned during the vice detox, the liver plays a central role in breaking down and eliminating excess estrogen. I had done my endocrine system a huge favor by jump-starting that organ first—a gesture that would have no doubt eased my withdrawal from the pill a lot better than the gluten-free chocolate chip cookies and red wine I had prescribed instead for my painful periods.

The one area that I still hadn't found a long-term solution for, though—and one that was still causing me anxiety a few months into my project—was birth control. I needed to address my needs in a more integrative way and come to terms with my new hormonal picture post-pill.

Coitus Interruptus

Charlie and I had been dating for long enough that we'd had some of the big trust conversations that come with exploring birth control methods beyond condoms. I was confident he wasn't bringing anyone or anything, aside from

Baron the Beagle, into our shared bed. But there were still big questions around what other options remained. I wasn't going to go back on the pill. And the idea of an implant like a copper IUD felt too invasive to try during a year dedicated to healing my body naturally. Who knew how my hawkish immune system would react to this semi-permanent foreign object?

The handful of my girlfriends who'd gone off (and stayed off) the pill seemed equally adrift in their search for alternatives. And the more openly I talked about my own conundrum, the more people admitted that they had been relying on their significant others to pull out.

"It's either the best birth control method ever, or I'm just infertile," one of them told me after a few glasses of wine. Another, who was still on the pill, just shook her head. "You guys are idiots."

I tended to agree. I had been told in eighth-grade sex ed that as soon as a penis enters your vagina, it can result in a pregnancy. I didn't need a middle school teacher to tell me that my life thereafter wouldn't necessarily look like an episode of *Gilmore Girls*. And yet, in 2011, 45 percent of American pregnancies were unplanned, this despite the fact that nearly half of those couples were using contraception at the time they conceived. If other forms of birth control are that fallible, why does withdrawal still carry the stigma of reproductive roulette?

Around this time, new research began circulating about coitus interruptus and the Interwebs seemed abuzz with the method's unspoken popularity. As the feminist journalist Ann Friedman wrote in *New York Magazine*, the pullout generation is made up of women who "buy organic kale and all-natural cleaning products, and so can't quite get down with taking synthetic hormones every day." Most are in committed relationships and therefore have already nurtured the degree of trust needed to cede that kind of control to a man. And many acknowledged some comfort in handing over the reins; it's stressful to be the lone watchdog guarding the hen house.

CONTRARY TO POPULAR BELIEF, pre-ejaculatory fluid is secreted by the Cowper's gland, not by the testicles. Like nature's Drano, this clear liquid cleans the urethra and provides safe passage for sperm released at ejaculation. The main risk is ensuring that there's no leftover semen present in the shaft from a prior roll in the hay. If the man has peed since the last time he ejaculated, in theory, that's sufficient to flush out the stragglers.

There are conflicting studies, however, on whether it's still possible for this fluid to contain sperm—most have too small a sample size to provide any definitive answer, and given the number of people googling it, the subject could benefit from more concrete research. Withdrawal advocates maintain that the occurrence is infrequent, if not impossible. In the largest study to date (twenty-seven subjects), all but one pre-ejaculatory sample contained fewer than twenty-three million sperm. While that sounds like a significant amount, counts this low correlated to just 2.5 percent of men whose partners conceived in less than one year.

There is, of course, still plenty of room for human error. I would presume the failure rates for coitus interruptus are largely due to misfires—a lack of male mastery over their own instruments—rather than a few measly sperm hanging out in the canal. It's a method that separates the men from the boys. And even for the former, it's probably one that's best practiced with a safety net before making it the sole method of contraception.

If used correctly, though—meaning the man pulls out before climax—data suggests that withdrawal has only a slightly higher failure rate than condoms (4 percent and 2 percent, respectively, with perfect use). And the rate for typical use, though high for both, doesn't differ greatly either. Which perhaps makes the case that relying on a man for either type of contraception is risky.

Despite these statistics, and even though I was wary of admitting it to others, as our relationship evolved and matured, we began slowly transitioning from condoms to the withdrawal method. Maybe that made me an idiot. But until I found a better system, I decided to put my trust in Charlie's ability to know his body well enough to prevent it from impregnating mine, and hope that the numbers were on my side.

The Fertile Window

As I was passively deliberating the contraception piece of my journey, an invite landed in my inbox for an evening dedicated to fertility awareness.

I showed up fairly clueless about what exactly this headline meant. It wasn't until I started listening to the presentation that I realized "fertility awareness" was a natural birth control method in and of itself, one that hadn't come up in conversations with girlfriends or Dr. A.

The talk was being given by Katinka Locascio, a trained doula and the founder of Earth & Sky Healing Arts, a center that offers fertility-based bodywork, along with consultations on how to chart your menstrual cycle.

As I listened to the presentation, I realized that for someone bingeing on health books like Honey Boo Boo at a pie-eating contest, I knew embarrassingly little about how my body conspired to make a mini me. I didn't know that an egg could only live for twelve to twenty-four hours. Or that the snail trail in my panties was, in fact, industrious cervical fluid designed to keep sperm alive inside a woman's body for up to five days. And I didn't realize that its changing viscosity was not random but, rather, tied to specific phases of my cycle.

Though the pullout method had been working for us so far, I was constantly paranoid about getting pregnant. Every time my period appeared, it felt like a small miracle. Just being told that I was fertile for less time than not each month made me feel better about the natural contraception method I was using. I was even more relieved when I saw withdrawal featured on Katinka's slide of available birth control methods. I became less so when I read the line item right below it: wild carrot seeds.

"What the hell is that?" I whispered to my friend, a health coach I'd run into in the lobby.

She giggled under her breath. "I've tried them."

"What?" I said, shocked.

"Yeah. I bought them from a man on the street in the East Village."

When taken orally after sex, she explained, the seeds can disrupt the implantation process. "My whole yoga studio started using them." She paused. "And then one girl got pregnant."

MAGICAL
WILD
CARROT
SEEDS

Later on, during a panel discussion, one fertility coach said that she always starts contraception conversations with her clients by asking them, "How tragic would it be if you got pregnant?" She then advised a method based on their answer and how able they were to execute on the various options.

I hoped that the yogi with the wild carrot seeds wouldn't have answered "very."

THE PRIMARY FORM of birth control Katinka, a fertility awareness method (FAM) educator, was there to discuss was menstrual cycle charting.

The practice, also known as the sympto-thermal method, relies on a woman monitoring and tracking various indicators of her daily fertility, allowing her to predict her fertile window.

"One of the biggest misconceptions, and the reason why charting may still be on the fringe, is that people think it's the same thing as the ineffective rhythm method," Katinka explained. "This is most certainly not the case. FAM requires more work but, when done properly, it is very effective—on par with the pill."

The rhythm method makes the false assumption that a woman has a consistent cycle. In theory, if you establish your past cycle length and abstain during the fertile window, you won't get pregnant. In reality, though, every woman's cycle is different from month to month—it can range anywhere from twenty-one to thirty-five days—and ovulation is always a moving target. Hence why abiding by the rhythm method is actual reproductive roulette.

Instead of trying to predict the window based on past cycles, the process of charting looks at several signs in the body on a day-to-day basis to confirm when you are actually fertile. Understanding the four phases of a woman's cycle—menstrual, follicular, ovulatory, and luteal—is essential for grasping how it works. And while I hoped that the practice would serve as a more reassuring birth control method than pulling out, I also realized that it was an important step in getting a better handle on my hormones.

Managing my blood sugar and reducing contact with endocrine disruptors had helped get my motherboard off the fritz. But if I wanted to help support my hormone levels throughout my cycle, I needed to know definitively where in my cycle I *was* at any given time.

With FAM, I could identify when I needed to double down on my birth control methods for extra protection and when to load up on tampons in anticipation of my flow. Using eco-minded condoms one

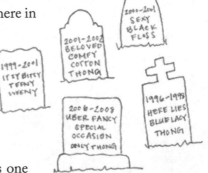

week out of the month didn't seem like as big of a drag. Plus, how many lacy pastel thongs would be saved if I had the ability to know if my period was about to hit when I got dressed in the morning?

On the subway ride home, I downloaded Kindara, a fertility awareness app, and entered the date of my last period. One four-dollar CVS thermometer later, and I was ready to begin charting.

There Will Be Blood

After Katinka's lecture, I turned directly to the seminal text of charting: Toni Weschler's *Taking Charge of Your Fertility*. Since the publication of her book two decades ago, Weschler has sparked a grassroots movement, offering generations of women the practical information they need to get a handle on their hormones. It was a fascinating refresher on my own anatomy, a deep dive I never got from sex ed, *Cosmo*, or conversations with girlfriends.

The efficacy of charting relies heavily on this type of body literacy and your ability to complete the following steps:

1. *Check cervical fluid throughout the day.* What I'd previously known as "discharge" is actually an incredibly vital part of a woman's fertility. The cervix is filled with glands, called crypts—fluid-filled hotel rooms that provide sperm a comfortable stay. Since an egg can only live for twelve to twenty-four hours, cervical fluid is essential for increasing the fertile window from one or two days (if a second egg gets released) to an average of eight. Typically, sticky cervical fluid begins appearing a few days after the end of your period, indicating that your fertile window has opened. As you approach ovulation, the amount of cervical fluid produced increases and its consistency becomes wetter, morphing from a creamy lotion into an elastic egg white. This is the key indicator for us pregnancy

avoiders that it's time to batten down the hatches and take down the sperm hotel's vacancy sign.

2. *Take waking temperature.* While cervical fluid is important for determining when the fertile window has begun, your basal body temperature (BBT)—taken first thing in the morning—is needed to confirm ovulation. During the first half of your cycle, your temperature plateaus at a lower range (usually below 98.0°F). After ovulation, your BBT rises sharply to create a better habitat for a potential bun in the oven and stays there for the rest of your cycle. A clear shift of two degrees or more, maintained for three days, confirms that ovulation has happened. Even if you're not using charting as a birth control method, your BBT also indicates where your hormones stand on a day-to-day basis. This is how you can confirm if you're not ovulating (a sign of PCOS), suffering from a luteal phase defect (which can be the hidden cause of repeat miscarriages), or experiencing adrenal issues. People with thyroid disorders tend to have temperature readings that push the low and high sides of the spectrum.

3. *Chart the data.* Mobile apps have made charting a whole lot easier than lugging a piece of graph paper with you every day to work or relying on the power of your own recall for the types of cervical fluid you observe throughout the day. Ideally, you want to check every time you go to the bathroom and record the consistency of what you find. Taking your temperature should happen first thing in the morning—and ideally at the same hour every day. Tracking these patterns relies on consistency, so if you oversleep, it should be noted. As I learned in my sleep experiments, your temperature rises as the morning goes on (thanks to melatonin levels falling with the first sign of light). Charting is yet another incentive to maintain the same waking time every day.

4. *Prevent pregnancy during the fertile window.* FAM can be up to 99.4 percent effective if executed perfectly and practiced with abstinence

during the fertile window, as religious incarnations, like natural family planning (NFP), advise. If using another form of contraception during that period of risk, the failure rate drops to the reliability of whatever barrier method you've chosen.

KNOWING THAT I would need to get a few cycles under my belt before I could establish my patterns and confidently rely on FAM for contraception, I dove into charting immediately, without the forethought to consult my significant other.

"Ugh, what are you doing," Charlie moaned from underneath the covers as my cheap thermometer bleated in a hostile key. 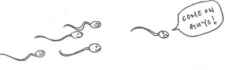 He looked bewildered as I gave him a muffled reply through clenched lips.

"I'm starting a new practice for keeping track of my fertility," I said, excitedly, once I had recorded my temperature. "Eventually, it will allow us to have sex without pulling out for part of the month."

Instead of mirroring my enthusiasm, Charlie looked even more alarmed than when my thermometer had roused him from sleep a few minutes earlier.

"You want to use the rhythm method?"

"No, no, no—this is different," I said, my voice revealing the self-righteous indignation of one who had just read five hundred pages on the subject. "It's science, babe."

"Oh, *science*," he replied sarcastically. "I thought that was how babies were made. My mistake."

It was too early in the morning to get into the intricacies of cervical crypts and follicle-stimulating hormones, so I simply replied, "For now, it's just something I'm doing for myself, okay?"

And it was true.

My friend, the fellow pullout practitioner, wasn't the only one questioning whether it was her own withering eggs or the withdrawal method that was responsible for her staying baby-free. As much as I didn't want to get pregnant right now, I also harbored the more nagging fear that I might never be able to. I had read about women who went off the pill in order to get pregnant, only to find that their fertility was in dire straits. For some, it took months to get their period back because of untreated PCOS. For others, extended use of the pill dried up their cervical crypts, leaving them without that essential fertile fluid. Maybe it was reading about these cases, or perhaps it was simply the unshakable creepiness of having been on artificial hormones for so long that made me wonder: *is anything even working down there?*

When I witnessed my first clear temperature shift two weeks later, the relief I felt made the initial charting annoyances seem like small potatoes. I knew I was ovulating. The cervical fluid in my sperm hotel was still intact (even if I didn't want anyone taking residence there). And on day 27, as I saw my morning temperature drop sharply, I knew immediately *there will be blood.*

Finding Your Flow

I was surprised at how quickly my charting practice became a new habit. I moved my thyroid medication next to my bed and took it as soon as I was done with my thermometer, which kept me on task with both mandatory morning practices. (I also learned to keep my earplugs in to help drown out the obnoxious beeps.)

There were a few logistical issues in the beginning, the biggest one being that Charlie and I lived on opposite sides of the city. This meant I had to plan ahead and remember to bring my thermometer with me when

I slept over. Since it's really the patterns that matter and not necessarily your temperature itself, using the same device consistently matters more than it being perfectly calibrated.

The more I charted, the more attuned I became to what was going on in my body from week to week.

Some of the exhaustion I used to attribute to a poor night's sleep or being "thyroid-y" appeared to be cyclical once I started paying attention— a result, usually, of the energy dip during the post-ovulation luteal phase. On days when going out with friends felt like a chore, it was comforting to know that I wasn't becoming a hermit, it was just my body telling me to rest and refuel for the time being.

There were weeks when I needed to honor my health, and times when I could get away with a little more hedonism. Perhaps the decision to wear gray sweatpants versus a cocktail dress, to sleep versus to socialize, didn't need to be so fraught. My hormones were very clearly calling the shots.

With three months' worth of charts behind me and just a few remaining in my wellness project, I wanted to use this new information to support my shifting energies—and create a more permanent system for integrating all of my new lifestyle practices according to my monthly flow.

For a road map, I turned to Alisa Vitti, the founder of FLOliving.com, a platform for integrative ways to resolve the root causes of period and fertility issues.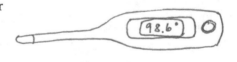

Vitti came up with her concept of Cycle Syncing™ the hard way after being diagnosed with PCOS in her early twenties. Dissatisfied with the doctors who told her she'd need to be on medication her whole life and would never be able to get pregnant, in the years following her diagnosis she began tailoring her diet, exercise, and lifestyle to her cycle. And it worked.

"Hormones get a bad rap for making women moody and unpredictable," says Vitti. In reality, though, their fluctuations are what give us our vitality, fuel our fertility, and bring our bodies into balance. "You have these distinct hormonal ratios that happen during each of the four phases of your menstrual cycle. Eating foods and selecting activities that optimize them ensures that you eliminate the common and unnecessary experience of PMS and period pain. You are designed hormonally to feel good in your body all month long!"

In her book, *WomanCode*, Vitti has a comprehensive chart of foods and activities that support the four phases. But she helped me make some generalizations by dividing my cycle into two parts.

Between the follicular and ovulation phases, your body needs additional support to metabolize estrogen. It's a perfect time to eat raw, sprouted, or fermented foods, and to take on high-impact activities like kickboxing, spinning, and other intense cardio. Even at work, you can use this extra energy to hit the ground running on new projects, go out into the world to meet clients, or beast some nagging tasks.

Once your body shifts into the second half of your cycle, the entrance of progesterone into the hormonal scene drives your focus inward. The need to nest during the post-ovulatory phase is deeply ingrained in our hormones. With all the focus on making enough progesterone, it's essential, according to Vitti, to eat foods that balance our blood sugar and give us the micronutrients we need to make that hormone in abundance. The luteal phase through menstruation is a good time for warming, cooked foods that are high in B vitamins and easier for the gut to process. It's also an opportunity for gentler exercise practices like Pilates and yoga that don't put additional demands on your metabolism and adrenals.

"Pushing yourself too hard in the gym when you're already struggling with exhaustion can cause stress and leave you feeling even more depleted," said Vitti. "Some women who train for triathlons or are really married to the same daily routine actually find that they can't lose that five to ten pounds because they're working against their hormonal needs with that type of exercise."

I wondered whether some of my boutique fitness experiences had been colored by my cycle. Perhaps I had popped my spin class cherry at the wrong time of the month.

For the next phase of my hormone experiments, I wanted to completely tailor my food intake and activities to my cycle. Though I wouldn't know exactly when ovulation hit until my temperature reading, my charts had been consistent enough that I could roughly sketch out the four phases on my Google Calendar. Already I saw that my week of bleeding was packed with work and social events that would require nights away from the comforts of my living room. I knew that I couldn't just become a recluse for two weeks every month, but for this experiment, I felt it was important to honor my body when it needed the most downtime.

With a few emails, I had rescheduled a class I was to teach and told a white lie to get out of a friend's cookbook launch party, knowing that with my impending morning cramps I would dread going anyway.

Ragtime

Six days later, when my alarm went off at seven a.m., I didn't even have to look at my thermometer to know that my moontime was upon me. The angry little man in my uterus was already having a tantrum, making it hard to justify getting out of bed.

In the past, I had always written off this day as my least productive of the month—the one that made me grateful to work from home, where I could spend prolonged stretches of time in the fetal positon audibly whimpering. But I was determined to give myself an attitude adjustment.

According to Vitti, the menstrual phase is an important interval for self-analysis and intuitive gut messages. So instead of dragging myself out from under the covers, as I had learned to do during sleep month, I settled in with my notebook.

Just a few months away from the end of my project, I was also wrapping up the third decade of my life. As I sat in bed, I tried to understand why contemplating my thirtieth birthday filled me with a feeling of impending doom. Was I berating myself for things I hadn't accomplished yet in my career? Areas of my wellness that I hadn't managed to solve? What dark places in my mind were still preventing my body from fully healing? Approaching a fork in the road tends to kick your intuition into overdrive. I wanted to follow my instincts at the time of the month when they were most accessible.

After an hour of journaling, the rest of the day was a low-key version of my usual routine. The only exception was lunch: instead of giving myself a break in the kitchen and ordering in something indulgent as a reward for my misery, I made myself an iron-rich bowl of kale and roasted beets with a sprinkle of torn nori strips.

Pop culture tells us the best cure for period cramps is a box of doughnuts and a Sandra Bullock rom-com marathon. While the latter might have some health benefits, your period is actually the time of the month when you most need nourishing whole foods and to avoid taxing an already turbulent hormonal system with sugar and caffeine (e.g., chocolate).

Per Alisa Vitti's recommendation, I rubbed clary sage essential oil—a natural remedy that's been shown in several studies to relieve cramps—on the area above my pubic bone. It felt like nature's IcyHot. I also restocked my cabinet below the sink with a box of organic cotton tampons.

Conventional cotton is one of the most toxic crops, using over 25 percent of the world's pesticides. Most tampons also use bleaching agents, synthetic fragrances to neutralize odor, and other chemicals. We know that these toxins can get passed through our skin, and they get absorbed even more quickly through the interior walls of the vagina, where there's no extra membrane for protection. Not only does this disrupt the delicate vaginal ecosystem, but it can cause even more inflammation and pain in the pelvis.

That night, instead of forcing myself to go out, I took an Epsom salt bath, slathered coconut oil on my bristly legs, pulled on my gray sweatpants, and curled up on the couch for a restorative night of watching Sandra's escapades in the Alaskan wilderness.

Sexual Healing

For a lot of women, it might seem silly to think about sex as a concrete part of your wellness plan. But like diet and exercise, it has a big impact on your ability to manage your hormone levels.

Sex is one of nature's best stress relievers, thanks to the oxytocin that's released during a romp under the covers. This seductive hormone not only triggers that warm, fuzzy feeling of attachment to the person panting below (or on top of) you but also helps balance ovulation, improve fertility, and slow down the aging process. And despite the fact that your hormones might not be compelling you to seek out sex at this time of the month, orgasms might just be better than Midol for menstrual cramps.

The key, according to Vitti, is to embrace the orgasmic plateau. When there's an absence of foreplay and climax is reached too quickly—thanks to an impatient partner or overstimulating vibrator—a woman doesn't get as many health benefits as she would if there was a sustained release of oxytocin.

"Fifteen minutes of self-pleasure with your hands is incredible medicine for your hormone balance, immunity, and moods," she said. This is true no matter where you are in your cycle, but certain phases might cause you to crave more sexual healing than others.

One study found that women who cheat on their husbands are much more likely to do so during ovulation. "If you're a single woman midway through her cycle, you may find yourself on a bar stool or a set of front steps you swore you'd never climb again," Mary Roach observed in her fascinating book *Bonk: The Curious Coupling of Science and Sex.* "Hormones are nature's three bottles of beer."

Men, whose hard-wiring is not dedicated to the multipronged art of growing a tiny human, are fertile (and potentially horny) 24/7. They are, however, biologically fine-tuned to sniff out our cyclical nuances. Several studies found that men are more drawn to the scent of a woman's perspiration while ovulating, versus at other times of the month.

Women on the pill, who don't ovulate, might not benefit from these unconscious forces of attraction. Mood swings and depression join a long list of symptoms, but another insidious one is the loss of libido. Some might argue that lifting the fear of pregnancy outweighs any dip in sex drive. And others, like my former self, simply never know what they're missing. It does bear asking the question, though: What's the point of going on birth control if you never want to have sex? If it could mean not putting yourself out there, or potentially giving yourself a pheromone handicap when you do?

Despite the best scientific intentions, bending our hormones to our will pulls at the delicate Darwinian threads that rule our fertility and desire. We are more primal than we realize. The laws of attraction might not be so fickle after all. Or at least, not in the ways that rom-coms had led me to believe.

I was glad that having a real cycle again allowed me to fully reap the rewards of sex as medicine. It was hard to do an accurate comparison of my pre- versus post-pill behavior, but I did know that since going off hormonal birth control and subsequently meeting Charlie, my desire had never been stronger. Perhaps it's that my pheromones had led me to the right match, or that ovulating again brought back my sex drive, or that love indeed conquers all, even an imperfect libido. Either way, all the oxytocin in my system was a welcome addition for my health and hedonism. And I didn't need an official experiment to convince me to get more of it.

The Sweet Spot

Even though I went kicking and screaming, going off the pill was a very necessary step that set the stage for all of my hormone experiments during this project. After all, you can't learn how to support your cycle if you don't have a cycle in the first place.

It took a lot more than a two-minute morning conversation to get my significant other on board with the idea of charting as birth control. Once Charlie understood FAM, though (and even corrected a friend who asked whether it was the rhythm method), it was a relief to have him more intimately involved in my fertility.

Safe sex means more than just contraception and consent. There's an element of communication that's fundamental to a relationship's success, inside and outside the bedroom. In this sense, charting was great for my sexual wellness. Even after Charlie downloaded my fertility app to his phone, it still forced us to constantly check in with each other.

The control I thought I had lost—the ability that artificial hormones gave me to plan ahead, skip periods, and know that I wouldn't get pregnant—I gained back. Instead of white pants surprises, I got a very clear red flag that my period was nigh and I had better run to CVS, prep the hot water bottle, and apologize to Charlie for snapping at him. Knowing where I stood in my cycle made it easier to understand the lure of different hormonal momentums. And it also gave me a window into how my thyroid was performing on a monthly basis, in between rounds of blood work.

While my temperature ranges remained fairly consistent, I noticed how the length of my cycle became longer when my thyroid was struggling and shorter on the one occasion that I increased my medication and accidentally dipped into hyperthyroid territory. It made me appreciate even more the power of my period as a canary in the coal mine, letting me know when something deep in my body was amiss.

FOR PEOPLE WITH AUTOIMMUNE DISEASE, it's especially important to choose your daily obligations wisely and set aside time to refuel. One of the tenets of Christine Miserandino's spoon theory is that people with a chronic illness only have so much energy to spend on the tasks of living. While healthy people may not feel the impact of something as minor as cooking dinner, ill or disabled people need to budget their reserves until the next opportunity to refill their well. I certainly understood this when I was at my sickest. So many of my self-care practices went down the tubes because I simply didn't have the vigor to execute them. But my

MENSTRUAL
wilted kale
sweet beets

FOLLICULAR
crunchy
romaine
creamy
avocado

roasted
root veg.
crispy
chickpeas

LUTEAL

raw
asparagus
spring onions

OVULATORY

cycle-syncing experiment helped me understand that for women, our energy reservoir operates on a monthly clock as well.

Before I started charting, I thought choosing to spend my Friday night in an Epsom salt bath instead of at a bar was just a part of getting older—a worrisome sign about where my capacity for fun was heading as I inched closer toward my thirtieth birthday.

But as I started paying more attention to my cycle, I realized it was more of an indication of the current week than the passing years. I learned when I could get away with less sleep, more cocktails, and plowing full steam ahead, and when I needed to pump the breaks on my social life to hibernate for menstrual winter. This experiment helped me feel less guilty about the occasional late night during the first half of my cycle, by helping me focus on staying closer to home during the times when my body needed it most. My periods didn't necessarily become less painful, but the misery was more contained. If I cared properly for myself on day one, I usually felt better the next morning rather than even more depleted.

Part of this was eating in tune with my hormonal appetites. I found it easiest to think of my cycle's four phases as mirroring the seasons, with the follicular phase and ovulation best suited to spring and summer fare, and the luteal phase and menstruation giving way to slow-cooked fall and winter comfort foods.

It was hard to pinpoint if any one ingredient did the trick, but getting more wholesome foods when my hormone levels were at their lowest did seem to direct my PMS roller coaster on a slightly less treacherous track than when I treated myself to wine and cookies. And it also helped my usually turbulent digestion during period week.

Through my research during these moon-sister experiments, I realized how important a healthy digestive system is for regulating your hormones, and vice versa—an unanticipated side effect of the pill is its impact on gut flora, making it harder to get the full nutritional value of your food.

I knew that syncing my cycle might only be doing a fraction of the good it could be if my microbiome was still out of balance. So that was exactly what I wanted to address next.

Learning to chart your fertility is a great first step to becoming more in tune with the moon-sister piece of your wellness puzzle. But there are plenty of other natural ways to regulate your rag time, practice safe sex, and honor your hormones.

1. *Manage your blood sugar.* As I learned during the vice detox, caffeine is problematic for women who are hormonally sensitive or compromised. "A good way to check if you're somebody who can tolerate it is to actually smell your pee," says Alisa Vitti. "If you have coffee and it smells normal, then you're better at breaking it down." Other hacks include going for a walk after a simple carb-heavy meal to immediately release some of the energy. (Get more tips on managing your blood sugar in chapter 1.)

2. *Restore nutrients post-pill.* When you're on hormonal birth control your body has a harder time absorbing vitamin B, magnesium, and zinc. These are not only essential nutrients for fertility, but also for your vitality. To improve your overall health while on the pill or transitioning off it, it's important to eat foods that boost these nutrient levels. If you aren't getting enough through food, ask your doctor if you need additional supplements.

3. *Don't forget about fat.* Women need to eat very differently in their childbearing years than they do in midlife, when they are often advised to eschew saturated fats and animal products. Subsisting on green salads alone deprives your body of essential fatty acids for hormone production, especially during menstruation.

While it's not wise to overdo it all month long, good-quality red meat is nourishing during your period because of all of the iron you lose from bleeding. For the rest of the month, oily wild fish, coconut oil, and omega-3-rich nuts and seeds stabilize your mood and energy. And bone broth (page 162) is one of the most restorative elixirs around.

4. *Use your moontime wisely.* Studies have shown that women's dreams are more frequent and vivid during the premenstrual and menstrual phases of their cycles. Once you can shed the attitude that your period is slowing you down, you can begin to honor this sacred time productively. Take those three days of pain and bloating to get quiet with yourself. Turn inward. Take Epsom salt baths, read, and put a hot water bottle (not a toxic heating pad) on your belly. Cancel plans. Relax. Sure, you might have to go to work. But try your best to get all of the fast-paced chores and tasks out of the way so you can do your most creative, visionary work during this time.

5. *Start following your cycle.* This chapter is by no means a complete guide to charting, and absolutely should not be used as your only resource if you're exploring using FAM as contraception. I recommend reading *Taking Charge of Your Fertility* or working with a coach or educator to help you through the process. Once you're ready, Kindara is one of the most comprehensive apps out there, and offers a community component to help you troubleshoot when you're confused.

6. *Don't stick toxic substances in your cooch.* Ingredients get absorbed through the vagina even more quickly than the skin because there's no barrier for protection. Disrupting the delicate vaginal ecosystem can also make you more susceptible to STDs. Opt for

organic, chemical-free tampons. (Check out brands, like LOLA, that offer a subscription service.) For sex toys, look for silicone, glass, metal, and ceramic, all of which are nonporous and are able to be sterilized. And remember, your hands are still the best toy around when it comes to feeding your hormones! Coconut oil is not only a practical addition to your kitchen and bathroom cabinets, it's also a great option to have in the bedroom as a natural lube. Just make sure you have separate jars; no one wants to be eating from the bedroom stash.

7. *A Brazil nut a day keeps the endocrinologist away.* Selenium is one of the most vital nutrients for thyroid health. It plays a critical role in the conversion of the primary thyroid hormone (T4) to the more bioavailable version (T3) and is essential for protecting against the toxicity of too much iodine in your diet. If you're a member of the Hashi Posse, eat three raw Brazil nuts a day. For an even more delicious option, make my Brazil Nut Pangritata (page 274) and add it to all your meals.

8. *Try a castor oil pack.* According to Acu Heidi and many healers before her, castor oil is the unsung hero of women's health. You can make an old-school pack by soaking a wool or cotton flannel in the oil and saran-wrapping it to your stomach, or use the modern option: a doggy wee-wee pad. When topped with a hot water bottle, these packs increase circulation through your entire pelvis and are said to help heal ovarian cysts and alleviate menstrual cramps. Truthfully, I've never been able to embrace this practice. But others find it to be the perfect activity for a quiet night on the couch, which is exactly what you want to do during your moon-time anyway, right?

SALADS FOR YOUR CYCLE

Luteal: Chili-Roasted Root Vegetables with Chickpeas, Tahini, and Brazil Nut Pangritata (page 274)

Menstrual: Marinated Kale with Tamari-Roasted Beets and Sesame Seeds (page 277)

Follicular: Grilled Romaine Hearts with Roasted Shallots, Artichoke Hearts, and Kefir Green Goddess Dressing (page 305)

Ovulatory: Shrimp and Asparagus Pesto Pasta Salad with Chives (page 308)

CHILI-ROASTED ROOT VEGETABLES WITH CHICKPEAS, TAHINI, AND BRAZIL NUT PANGRITATA

Serves 4

The luteal phase is when a woman's body benefits most from natural sugars and easy-to-digest cooked foods. The warming spices in this salad aid in digestion, and the selenium-packed Brazil nuts act as a complete thyroid supplement. Pangritata is essentially poor man's Parmesan. Back in the day when money was tight in the old country, Italian peasants would fry up coarsely chopped bread crumbs with other cheap staples like garlic and herbs and serve the mixture over pasta instead of grated cheese. Brazil nuts add a similarly delicious crunch to these sweet roasted vegetables and keep the pangritata gluten-free.

....

1 large sweet potato (1 pound), cut into 1-inch cubes

4 small carrots ($^1/_2$ pound), cut into 1-inch pieces

4 small parsnips ($^1/_2$ pound), peeled and cut into 1-inch pieces

5 tablespoons olive oil

1 teaspoon cumin

1 teaspoon chili powder

$^1/_2$ teaspoon ground cinnamon

$1^1/_2$ teaspoons sea salt

One 15-ounce can chickpeas (about 2 cups cooked)

$^1/_3$ cup Brazil nuts, pulsed in the food processor or finely chopped

2 garlic cloves, minced

$^1/_4$ cup tahini paste

2 tablespoons freshly squeezed lemon juice

1 tablespoon finely chopped fresh parsley, for garnish

1. Position the racks in the upper and lower thirds of the oven and pre-heat the oven to 425°F. Line two rimmed baking sheets with parchment paper.

2. In a large mixing bowl, combine the sweet potato, carrots, parsnips, 3 tablespoons olive oil, cumin, chili powder, cinnamon, and 1 teaspoon salt. Toss until well coated in the oil and spices.

3. Arrange the veggies in an even layer on the prepared baking sheets. Roast for 20 minutes, then remove the pans and add the chickpeas. Return the pans to the oven, swapping the top one to the bottom, and cook for another 20 minutes, or until the vegetables are nicely browned and caramelized.

4. While the root veggies are roasting, make the pangritata: Heat the remaining 2 tablespoons of olive oil in a small skillet. Add the nuts and garlic and cook over medium heat until fragrant and lightly browned, about 3 minutes. Season with salt and set aside.

5. In a small mixing bowl, whisk together the tahini, lemon juice, and ½ teaspoon salt until a thick paste forms (culinary magic!). Add ¼ cup of water (or more) and stir until the sauce is the consistency of ranch dressing.

6. Transfer the roasted veggies to a serving plate, drizzle with the tahini sauce, and garnish with the Brazil nut pangritata and parsley.

HEALTHY HEDONIST TIPS

The tough skin on veggies is often the healthiest part. For example, potato skins have far more fiber, antioxidants, iron, potassium, and B vitamins than the pale flesh underneath. (Another rule of vibrancy!) I leave the skin on the carrots and sweet potatoes but peel the parsnips since the outside can be slightly bitter.

MARKET SWAPS

Any root veggies will work here, just make sure you have 2½ pounds total. Delicata and butternut squash are great options in the fall. To make
this a main course salad, use 5 ounces of peppery arugula as a bed for the
veggies. If part of your batch-cooking session, simply keep the salad
greens and tahini sauce separate and assemble to order. The pangritata
can keep for up to 2 weeks in the fridge and also tastes wonderful sprin-
kled on top of soup or scrambled eggs.

MARINATED KALE WITH TAMARI-ROASTED BEETS AND SESAME SEEDS

Serves 2 to 4

I make a version of this salad pretty much every time I do a batch-cooking session. Ordinary lettuce leaves get soggy and sour if you dress them in advance, but kale? Be still my basic heart, it only gets better. *Don't be afraid to add an avocado rose as the cherry on top right before you serve.*

....

3 medium beets (about ³/₄ pound), scrubbed

3 tablespoons olive oil, divided

¹/₂ teaspoon sea salt

2 tablespoons tamari

1 tablespoon sesame seeds

1 bunch of Tuscan kale (also known as lacinato, dinosaur, or cavolo nero)

2 tablespoons freshly squeezed lemon juice

1 garlic clove, minced

1 teaspoon sesame oil

1 avocado, thinly sliced (optional)

1. Preheat the oven to 425°F. Line a rimmed baking sheet with parchment paper.

2. Dice the beets into 1-inch cubes and toss them with 1 tablespoon olive oil and the salt on the prepared baking sheet. Arrange in an even layer and roast until lightly browned, about 15 minutes. Remove from the oven and add 1 tablespoon tamari and the sesame seeds. Toss until well coated, spread evenly, and return to the oven. Cook another 10 minutes, or until the beets are very tender.

3. Meanwhile, remove the thick stem from the center of the kale leaves and discard. Stack the leaves in a pile, roll them up like a cigar, and slice thinly. Set aside in a large mixing bowl. Add the remaining 2 tablespoons of olive oil, the remaining 1 tablespoon of tamari, the lemon juice, garlic, and sesame oil to the kale and toss until the leaves are very well coated in the dressing. Don't be afraid to manhandle it a little!

4. Top the salad with the roasted beets and avocado, if using.

HEALTHY HEDONIST TIPS

If you're eating this recipe during your week of menstruation (as you definitely should), feel free to add some iron-rich grass-fed steak or lamb to make it a main course salad, and to help replenish your iron reserves.

MARKET SWAPS

Any type of kale will work, but I prefer Tuscan or lacinato for raw preparations as the smooth leaves are more naturally tender and require less massaging. Instead of olive oil, you can sub blood sugar–balancing melted coconut oil. Just make sure to serve the salad at room temperature, since the oil can solidify when cold. Dried cranberries or sliced apples for sweetness is another tasty addition.

EATER'S DIGEST

GUT CRITTERS AND THE SCOOP ON MY POOP

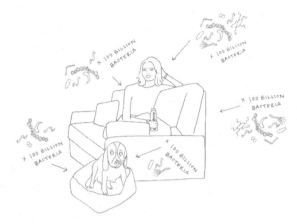

*On replanting my gut garden and making
my digestive system my new BFF.*

During my early years of autoimmune denial, my stomach tried very hard to get my attention. Every meal was met with dissent, as if the underappreciated workers of my digestive system had gathered with picket signs in my alimentary canal. Taking gluten out of my diet years earlier had helped set things right to some extent, but even after getting my food choices under control during my clean-eating experiments, my digestion still sometimes got a little janky without my really understanding why.

Part of improving conditions in the gut is catering to the palates of its many inhabitants: the hundred trillion bacteria that make up our microbiota. As my project progressed, more and more research emerged on the role the microbiome plays in warding off sickness, losing weight, and maintaining good mental health. And the findings challenged the

long-held notion that germs should be met with an iron-clad Trump im-
migration policy. These visitors, it seems, just might hold the key to
achieving long-term good health.

Studies have shown that the balance of bacteria on our skin, in our
nether regions, and, most notably, throughout our twenty-five-foot-long
intestinal tract, can either protect us from or propel us toward a variety of
"modern plagues" such as obesity, depression, and, especially, autoimmune
disease, which might strike some of you as counterintuitive.

Having a compromised immune system can make you acutely paranoid about the pathogens lurking in the outside world. Over the course of
my project, discovering all the toxic dangers in my environment just
fanned the flames of these fears. I needed to get a better handle on the
immune-gut connection. If my dietary improvements thus far hadn't
been enough to recruit new members to my stomach's citizen army, what
other lifestyle changes did I still need to make? For this set of challenges,
I wanted to get more comfortable with my critters.

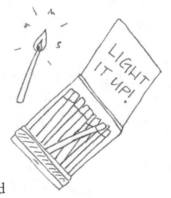

IRONICALLY, it may have been one of
these very critters that got me into my
big health mess in the first place.

The causes of autoimmune disease
are still fairly mysterious, but medical
legend has it that there's usually a trigger. As Heidi put it, most people spend
years accumulating imbalances—adding tinder to the box—but it takes
an emotional or physical event to light the match and set the whole fucker
on fire.

Before I started this project, I was still a little hazy on what sparked
that fateful flame, but there was no question about *when* it happened.

The summer after I graduated from college, my mother and I took a trip to Morocco. She'd lived there in her twenties, and it had been over a decade since she'd been back to visit friends. As my generous gift for making it through four years of poli-sci essays and beer pong, she took me along for two weeks of gorging on lamb tagines, hiking through the Atlas Mountains, and haggling for ethnic furnishings for my first New York City apartment.

That was the plan, at least.

In reality, I spent most of my time in Fez curled up in a ball on the *riad*'s bathroom floor with my cheek pressed against the turquoise mosaic tiles. It seemed that the figurative travel bug I had caught in college— which had taken me across another continent before I met up with my mother—had graduated into a very real critter in my intestines by the time I reached North Africa.

I eventually regained enough strength to make it out into the winding corridors of the medina but I never really recovered. My stomach was never the same after the trip. What was once an iron cauldron for Third World street meats and strip mall all-you-can-eat sushi became as sensitive as a saucepan of untempered eggs over a high flame.

I was diagnosed with Hashimoto's six months after returning stateside.

I didn't know enough at the time to connect the dots to my recent episode of traveler's tummy, but as I have come to understand, the health of our microbiome is irrevocably tied to our general immunity.

Since outside invaders primarily enter through the nose and mouth, the body's first line of defense is in the digestive tract. Seventy percent of our immune cells reside beneath the intestinal lining and rely heavily on their friends, your good bacteria, to function properly.

I like to picture these immune T cells as burly, aggressive bouncers at da club. Without a nod from the door girl with the clipboard, they would have no idea that the guy with the faux hawk was a member of One Direction and not just some other entitled douche bag trying to elbow his way to the front of the line. In other words, if the good bacteria weren't there to regulate, visitors who should be ushered into your gut's VIP area might instead get punched in the face.

Not only do resident bacteria help prevent your overprotective T cells from going into overdrive, they also provide their own line of defense against dangerous invaders before your immune cells even get involved.

For starters, they produce stomach acid.

Those of us who have watched one too many Prevacid commercials may not realize that the harsh pH of our stomach is actually very necessary for making sure bad bacteria doesn't survive the first leg of the digestive labyrinth. If they do make it to the intestines (perhaps a result of popping one too many proton-pump 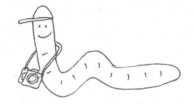 inhibitor pills, like Prevacid), your good bacteria then emit their own "antibiotics," which stop foreign pathogens in their tracks and prevent them from taking up permanent residence.

Where had this symbiotic army been when I was in Morocco? Well, in a gut already ravaged by four years of activities that damage gut flora—heavy alcohol consumption, birth control pills, sleepless All-Night Tuesdays, fat-laden Chicken Finger Fridays—a little bad bacteria could do a lot of damage.

Once the invaders make their way past the stomach, they unleash their own special brand of toxins with the fury of Kanye West at a Taylor Swift concert. These attacks weaken the intestinal walls in the process, essentially spraying tear gas onto the dance floor and forcing innocent bacterial bystanders to flee.

My stomach bounced back to a semi-functional place after I returned home, but deep in my gut, an ongoing battle of good and evil was being waged. As the war quietly continued underground, my good bacteria slowly receded, their lines of defense crumbled, and my immune cells lost their masters of command.

No boy band member or gluten protein would ever be truly safe again.

Bacterial Breeding Ground

It took a much more recent invasion for me to see just how out of balance my microbes still were.

Around the time of our one-year anniversary, Charlie and I discovered we had a parasite. Now, this is not a cute turn of phrase the way some couples say "We're pregnant." No—we shared an intestinal bug as one shares chlamydia.

Charlie had brought his own set of gut baggage to the relationship. In college, his stomach issues were so bad, he'd ended up in the emergency room on more than one occasion, yet none of the gastroenterologists could figure out what was wrong with him. As a shot in the dark, they decided to remove his appendix.

Surprisingly, the surgery helped, at least for a few years. But by the time I wandered into his life, Charlie's stomach had become unpredictable again—even more so than my own. In the same way a CIA operative scans the room for exits and blind spots, Charlie had developed an internal GPS for locating the nearest restroom at all times. His issues were never so severe that they landed him back in the hospital, but they were enough of a problem that long car trips became a source of constant anxiety.

Being a meddlesome significant other, I had taken to using my acupuncture sessions with Heidi to talk through Charlie's ailments. When I mentioned he'd improved after the vestigial organ removal, it immediately sparked a theory.

"Sounds like a parasite," she said. "The appendix can be an incubator for good bacteria, but that also means it can incubate other shit. They could have gotten rid of a whole colony of critters by removing it, but the fact that he's having some of the same symptoms says to me that whatever frenemy he caught has started to take hold again."

Both Charlie and I had been tested for parasites after our respective tummy traumas and come up negative, but it's not uncommon for them to go unnoticed in stool samples; it's much better to seek them out in their home, the intestinal wall. Which is how I found myself on Dr. C's metal table after he succeeded in ferreting out the bug in Charlie's gut.

"Don't worry—he has small hands," Charlie teased before I left for my appointment.

Was this the crowning achievement of intimacy?

Dr. C's office was lined with diplomas and emeritus robes, which, combined with his white hair and calm demeanor, gave him the air of having multiple lifetimes under his belt—the Dumbledore of the infectious disease world.

As he began the procedure, my mind wandered back to my birth control conundrum. I'd been so careful to use protection during the early stage of our relationship. Who knew there were things to worry about aside from pregnancy and STDs?

"I didn't realize that you could pass bad bacteria back and forth," I said, making casual small talk.

"Oh, it's very common with couples," Dr. C replied, matter-of-factly. "Let's just say that when two people love each other very much and they go to bed together, they tend to touch each other all over."

I was grateful to be facing the wall, as my face contorted into a cringe. No one wants to think about the time Dumbledore spends sans his wizarding robes.

That afternoon, after he'd examined my sample on a slide, Dr. C called with the results.

"It's a common amoeba, *E. histolytica*," he said. "In Latin, that means 'tissue cutting.' It can be pretty placid if you have a good immune system but dangerous if you're a malnourished child in Africa or a chemo patient." He advised that Charlie and I start antiparasitics immediately. Hopefully, they'd rid the bugs from both our systems over the next two weeks.

"Don't expect to feel completely back to normal for a few months, though," said Dr. C. "It takes time for any part of the body to heal."

Back home, Charlie and I immediately began debating the origin of this shared parasite. Though I wanted to blame him, it seemed more likely that we had each brought something to the table that created a breeding ground for bad bacteria in our guts.

Missing Microbes

While learning that I had a parasite was disconcerting, in some ways I felt like I had found the answer I'd been searching for through months of wellness experiments and years of testing.

Many of my symptoms—mainly the bad skin—had gotten considerably worse as soon as Charlie and I started dating. At the beginning of the relationship, I had plenty of logical explanations: the increasing presence of bacon, eggs, and potatoes in my diet; my dwindling sleep reservoir; the dog hair on my pillow. But having my gut's ecosystem rattled by bad bacteria seemed to explain everything. And it was something I could actually fix.

Despite Dr. C's cautioning that healing could take months, Charlie and I both experienced a digestive renaissance within a few weeks of treatment. Not only did my stomach seem less irritable overall, but for the first time since I was diagnosed with Hashimoto's, my vitamin B_{12} and thyroid hormones were in the numerical vicinity of a healthy person's. I had seen some improvements in my blood work throughout my project, but nothing like this. When I got the most recent tests back, I had to do a double take to make sure the lab hadn't accidentally given me someone else's results.

Could a parasite have been the culprit all along? Had Gloria the Healer's diagnosis of an overgrowth in one of my organs been right after all? Perhaps my living room was not the only space that had been furnished with Moroccan keepsakes all these years.

All I knew was that my body was finally back on the rails again. Nine months into my year of wellness, I was actually starting to feel like I was healed.

TWO WEEKS LATER, I once again found myself cheek-to-bathroom tiles, my body violently purging itself of the ceviche I'd eaten at dinner. Charlie was also in bad shape, which made sharing a bathroom only slightly less harrowing than after our night of cheap tequila at the electronic music concert.

We had shared appetizers with another couple, yet only the two of us had come down with food poisoning. As Charlie and I learned the hard way, your microbiome doesn't differ from most world nations under attack; when you kill off the innocent and decimate infrastructure, it creates a perfect environment for an insurgency.

Such is the catch-22 of antibiotics.

There's no denying that the discovery of penicillin forever changed modern medicine for the better. But with these advances there have been some serious unanticipated consequences. Research has shown that people who take many courses of antibiotics over time are typically sicker, have immune systems that can no longer distinguish between friend and foe, and show a variety of other deficiencies as a result.

The process of building your microbiome begins at birth. As newborns pass through the vaginal canal, they're colonized on the spot by their mother's bacteria. C-section babies (now one in three births in the United States) miss out on this initial inoculation, which might explain why they go on to have much higher risks for allergies, obesity, and auto-immune diseases.

I hardly blame my current condition on the fact that I came into this world through my mother's abdomen instead of her vagina. If it hadn't been for that emergency extraction, I wouldn't even be here to complain about the state of my gut. But I do see how leapfrogging over this essential biological process—coupled with immediate antibiotic treatment and a diet of microbe-free baby formula—could lead to a fragile and anemic microbiome.

Broad-spectrum antibiotics kill protective and pathogenic bacteria alike. In fact, bad bacteria are notoriously harder to decimate in an antibiotic assault, essentially giving the surviving few the keys to the kingdom.

So how do you escape this vicious cycle? When it came to ridding our systems of the amoeba, did we really have a choice?

Bugs over Drugs

About a month after the parasite discovery, I found myself in an amphitheater listening to Dr. Robynne Chutkan wax poetic about the joys of being, in her words, a "doo doo doctor."

A traditional gastroenterologist by training, Chutkan's practice, the

Digestive Center for Wellness in Washington, DC, has become increasingly integrative since she began to focus on the role of the microbiome.

"Knowing what we do now, I think putting kids (or adults, for that matter) on antibiotics to treat acne, sometimes for years, is malpractice," she said, looking straight into the camera, as if staring down her prescription-happy peers. "We know that five days of a broad-spectrum antibiotic removes a third of your gut bacteria. Your skin might clear up in the short term, but often people develop deeper, more cystic acne. They switch antibiotics. They become resistant. And no one is really thinking of the downstream effects. We may actually be creating real diseases like Crohn's and MS through our overzealous use of antibiotics."

When the crowd attending the wellness conference dispersed for lunch, I practically pounced on her.

Dr. Chutkan nodded and listened politely as I relayed my recent gut troubles. Her talk had given me a resurgence of guilt, this time of the microbial variety. I needed her to tell me that I had done right by my body by taking the meds for my parasite and that the collateral damage couldn't have been helped.

But she was having none of that.

"When my patients ask me how they know if it's appropriate to use an antibiotic, I sort of joke and say: when death is imminent," Dr. Chutkan replied in between bites of her woody kale salad. "That might be an unreasonably high threshold. But I explain that when you have a cold, it's usually a viral illness. The antibiotic isn't even effective and it's doing a lot of damage."

"What about cases of traveler's stomach, though?" I asked.

"Well, certainly if there's a fever, blood, or serious dehydration involved, that's what we have medication for. It's really the unnecessary, ongoing courses of antibiotics I find so troubling."

The average American child takes one course of antibiotics a year, primarily for minor illnesses. Dr. Chutkan explained that in exchange for this short-term comfort—the relief from a sinus infection, a temporary clearing of acne, the slaying of a bad stomach bug—we make a dangerous trade.

As I looked back on my gut landscape, I realized how much damage I had probably done over the years with the half-dozen antibiotics prescribed by my dermatologist. Perhaps that was all it took for my bad bacteria to take hold again or join forces with Charlie's.

"Pills can be lifesaving," Dr. Chutkan emphasized. "But watchful waiting, while you allow your body to heal and recover, is sometimes the smarter approach. At least for your microbes. We'd all be better off if we learned to be a little more uncomfortable."

While antibiotics are the biggest threat, many other over-the-counter and prescription drugs also damage the gut, said Dr. Chutkan. Antacids and proton pump inhibitors change the pH of the stomach, breaking down that first wall of defense. Nonsteroidal anti-inflammatory drugs (NSAIDs) injure the intestinal lining, causing bacteria to translocate more easily. Birth control and hormone replacement therapies create estrogen levels that threaten the microbial ecosystem, leading to chronic candida and subsequent digestive issues.

I had been better about not popping Aleve, an NSAID, since my back problems subsided, and now when I had a headache, I turned to a glass of water first to see if that helped. But when I felt intense discomfort, like that bout of recent food poisoning, I reverted to my old habits of reaching for a pill to ease my symptoms.

Dr. Chutkan also suggested that while I may have gotten rid of my amoeba by drowning my gut in antiparasitics, not taking the time to re-plant all the good species I wiped out in the process left my system that much more vulnerable (hence the food poisoning). As I self-consciously finished my bison burger and sweet potato fries, I made a silent vow to do a better job feeding all of those indentured house elves in my gut's basement and stop blasting them with medication every time I experienced pain.

Minding my meds and eating clean was only half the battle, though. As Dr. Chutkan told me, I would also have to learn to live dirtier.

Hair of the Dog

As I thought about the trillions of bacteria already inhabiting my body, outnumbering my own cells three to one, I knew I had to loosen my grip on my "live clean" protocol.

The first part meant not over-washing my hands with antibacterial soap and getting rid of all the remaining toxic cleaning products in my home. I'd already replaced my harsh skin care with simple naturals, started shopping locally for pesticide-free vegetables that still had dirt from the farm on them, and filtered out harmful ingredients like chlorine from my tap and shower water—chemicals that kill delicate microbes on your skin and in your gut—but had yet to make the green transition with all the other bottles that kept my apartment spic and span.

In a city like New York, it's impossible to escape the grit and grime of everyday living. For us "lifers," this is a love-hate relationship. We love the smells, the buzz, the humanity. But at the end of the day, we're also happy to retreat to our cocoons of cleanliness and quiet—the sanctuaries we've established with our own chosen members of humanity, and their own special smells.

My *own* filth I was relaxed about—especially the types I found most annoying to eradicate, like rings around the toilet bowl or the crevices of the mirror that were forever splattered with toothpaste. It was the residue from the city below that I tried not to bring home with me. Mail and newspapers never got plopped on my kitchen countertops, and neither did my grocery receipts, which I learned were coated in BPA plastic.

Shoes came off right inside the door, and if those shoes were flip-flops, I'd take my grimy toes straight to the bathroom for a sponge bath.

I didn't realize the extent of my sanitary standards until a hairy, slobbering out-side visitor threatened my cocoon.

The first night Baron the Beagle spent in my apartment— for a weekend-long experiment in cohabitation on my turf— my reaction was so visceral that it caught me off guard. I had known the hair and dirt would be a problem. I didn't love it all over everything at Charlie's place. But I had 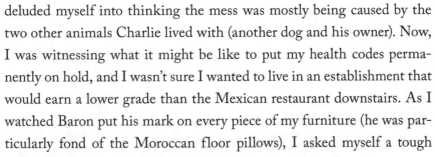 deluded myself into thinking the mess was mostly being caused by the two other animals Charlie lived with (another dog and his owner). Now, I was witnessing what it might be like to put my health codes perma-nently on hold, and I wasn't sure I wanted to live in an establishment that would earn a lower grade than the Mexican restaurant downstairs. As I watched Baron put his mark on every piece of my furniture (he was par-ticularly fond of the Moroccan floor pillows), I asked myself a tough question: was this germaphobia or was it really latent commitment phobia in disguise?

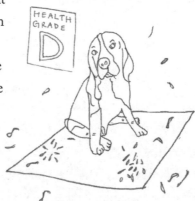

Meanwhile, I had never seen Charlie so happy, playing house with the three of us under the same roof. The boys returned home after a few days but the experience left some lasting doubts along with the white strands that now covered all of my area rugs.

Rewilding

It was clear that adjusting to living dirtier at home would take some time. But as I proceeded into Phase 2 of my microbiome experiment, I learned that Baron the Beagle might play a more important role in my health than I realized.

"In conservation biology, 'rewilding' means the introduction of species into areas where they've become extinct, with the goal of returning to a more natural and balanced existence," Dr. Chutkan wrote in her book *The Microbiome Solution.*

For humans, rewilding our guts also takes a little help from the outside world. And who are the best rewilding agents around? Yup. Dogs.

In support of the hygiene hypothesis, studies have shown that as the amount of concrete and glass in a community increases, so too does the risk of developing allergies and asthma. By sheltering ourselves in vehicles and office buildings—our cocoons of cleanliness—we miss out on an entire realm of microbes. On the other hand, households who drag in environmental detritus—like, say, fur that has been in contact with a fire hydrant—increase the immunity of their families by maximizing their exposure to all matters of microbial diversity. In fact, children who grow up with furry friends have far fewer instances of allergies and asthma than their dog-less peers.

Who knew that the secret weapon for my immune system had been perched on the couch all along, waiting to inoculate my face with his tongue?

Getting comfortable with a bit more dirt in my life was one thing; getting my hands dirtier in the first place was a different challenge. I didn't have a garden bed out back to

IMMUNITY

benefit from the rich soil. Nor did I really have the free time to wander barefoot every day in the grass of a nearby park. And with "real nature" at least a forty-five-minute train ride away, it seemed that for this piece of my challenge I would have to bring nature to me.

Dr. Chutkan suggests simply opening your windows as a baby step if you can't spend more time outside, and also filling your house with plants for additional exposure.

Both seemed fairly easy to accomplish. I didn't have a whole lot of shelf or counter space in my small studio, but I found a wall-mounted unit designed especially for easy-to-maintain indoor plants like succulents. They weren't as lauded for their air-purifying abilities as some other varieties (I'm looking at you, English ivy!), but if *Shark Tank* had invested in this aesthetically pleasing vertical garden, why shouldn't I?

The cheapest and easiest way, of course, to bring nature home with me was to welcome a furry creature inside. For the sake of my microbiome (not to mention the sake of my relationship), I realized I needed to mentally rebrand Baron the Beagle as a health bonus instead of a barrier. I would stop washing my hands every time I pet him. I would let him mouth-kiss with abandon. And I would try not to freak out when I used those same dirty hands to fish stray strands of fur out of my homemade fish stew.

Eating for Two Trillion

I still had my doubts about how getting dirtier would translate in New York City. The biggest conundrum of my new protocol was hand washing.

I knew I was supposed to avoid antibacterial agents at all costs. But out in the real world, that was next to impossible. Everywhere from a fancy restaurant on Fifth Avenue to the airport bathroom at JFK used antibacterial foaming soaps. This left me paralyzed. Was I supposed to use it and kill off all the good skin microbes I had fostered from my dog petting? Or just rely on hot water and hope it would be enough to ward off any subway pole pathogens on my fingers before I mindlessly cleaned potato chip grease off of them with my mouth?

Dr. Chutkan recommended the latter, unless I was visiting a particularly scummy bathroom with a high volume of foot traffic. I did my best to heed her protocol, but it was hard to shed the ick factor overnight.

Every morning when I opened my window to let in some "fresh" microbial-infused air and was hit by the warm fumes from the buses outside, I wondered: Without a grassy backyard, are we city dwellers destined to have depleted microbiomes? Or does riding public transportation in close proximity to someone coughing into their sleeve make our immune systems stronger?

I didn't understand how residue from the concrete jungle could be good for my microbes in the same way a frolic through the woods was. But perhaps people who live surrounded by nature are missing out on the microbial diversity that I experience every day on the crowded L train. At least that's what I decided to keep telling myself.

To measure my progress, I ordered a microbiome sequencing kit from uBiome and sent off a sample. The results would tell me how my gut's bacterial makeup stacked up against other demographics and, over time, to myself. A monthly subscription meant I could retest again after a few weeks of my new gut-conscious lifestyle to see if the changes had an impact.

For the last leg of my rewilding challenge I knew I needed to supplement my efforts by being smarter about what I was actually putting in my gut.

And "supplement" seemed like the operative word in terms of where to begin.

. . .

IN THE LAST SEVERAL YEARS, the probiotics market has skyrocketed into a thirty-billion-dollar global industry. These pills promise to deliver billions of organisms to the bed of your gut garden, along with any number of health benefits from weight loss to reduced risk of heart disease. While I knew that improving my microbiome might deliver on some of these claims, I was wary of which bottles in the vitamin aisle actually contained real bacteria instead of just snake oil.

One of the general misconceptions about probiotics is that these bottled bugs join your existing bacteria and take permanent residence in the gut. This is a myth that Erica and Justin Sonnenburg, the husband-and-wife power couple behind Stanford University's Department of Microbiology and Immunology, want to dispel.

"Probiotic bacteria are transient visitors," said Justin. "They serve as 'dummies' that allow the immune system to fine-tune its response to more dangerous microbes."

When I sat down with the Sonnenburgs in their home by way of Skype, they were haloed by a black-and-white framed print hanging in the background—a Keith Haring–style portrait of bacteria that looked like a smattering of overlapping cheese curls. That's commitment to the cause, I thought.

On the subject of probiotic pills, the Sonnenburgs admitted that efficacy is difficult to test. Because each of us has a different microbiota—more unique in its complexity than a fingerprint—there's no such thing 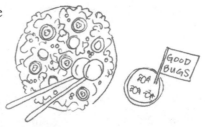 as a one-size-fits-all solution. One combination could work in one individual but not another. For this reason, the Sonnenburgs recommend eating lacto-fermented foods—like yogurt, kefir, sauerkraut, kimchi, and kombucha—as they contain the most bacterial diversity. Adding a variety of these foods to your diet gives you the opportunity to hedge your bets in a way that no one pill ever could.

I was also curious about the newly emerging term "prebiotic." Many probiotic companies now sell pills with this built-in bonus that claims to increase the effectiveness of the bacteria once it reaches your gut.

The scientists gave me a little smirk, an expression that in less polite people would have manifested as an eye roll.

"Really the whole vegetable aisle should have a big sign on it saying 'prebiotics,'" said Erica. Complex carbs with insoluble fiber make up the cuisine our resident bacteria crave most. Think basically any legume, whole grain, and, yes, the whole vegetable aisle. They don't feed the probiotics, per se. Rather, vegetables are a central part of a good gut diet. Without them, you're not giving your resident bacteria any food to survive on. In other words, if you're subsisting on actual cheese curls and hamburgers, probiotic pills at a dollar a pop might be a waste of money. What's the point of dousing your garden with expensive fertilizer if no one is going to water the plants?

One of the reasons edible probiotics like vegetable-based kimchi and kraut are so effective is that they cross-train your system with new transient bacteria and feed the existing community at the same time. It's like giving your gut an all-inclusive spa weekend at Canyon Ranch versus a day pass to Bally Total Fitness followed by dinner at McDonald's.

Besides feasting on fiber, the second good gut rule of thumb is to limit meat and saturated animal fat. In the simplest terms, red meat messes with your bacterial metabolism, producing dangerous compounds that contribute to the risk of stroke and heart attack. More worrisome, though, is that 80 percent of our country's antibiotic production goes toward livestock. While you can choose to take or leave your doctor's prescription slip, eating factory-farmed meat exposes your gut to a cloud of microbial tear gas whether you like it or not.

Feeding your beneficial bacteria a plant-based diet is important for maintaining their ranks, and it also prevents them from feasting off the next best thing: you. As the Sonnenburgs explain in their book, *The Good Gut: Taking Control of Your Weight, Your Mood, and Your Long-Term Health*, when your bacteria are deprived of fiber, their alternate food source is the mucous lining of the intestines, which leads to immune dysfunction and leaky gut disease.

I was already squarely in the less meat, more veg camp thanks to my anti-inflammatory eating conversion, which still inspired me to go plant-based for most of my meals and invest in antibiotic-free organic options when I did eat animals. And thanks to my hormone experiments, I was more in tune with when my body actually craved red meat—a few times a month during menstruation. It was a relief to know that my past challenges lined up with a good gut diet. All I needed to do going forward was add more fermented foods to the mix.

Proof in the Pudding

While I waited for my uBiome results to come back, I monitored my daily progress with a poop log.

People get squeamish about toilet talk. And yet, our bowel movements remain the best way to gauge how our digestive systems are performing on a daily (and sometimes hourly) basis. I was now paying more attention to my cervical fluid to know where my hormones stood. So during my gut challenge, to get the same data for my digestion, I tried to take stock before flushing those valuable clues down the toilet.

Paying attention to my BMs indicated that one probiotic a day might just keep the gastroenterologist away. I noticed that when I made a concerted effort to ingest one of the four Ks—kombucha, kefir, kraut, or kimchi—my system ran much smoother. And adding extra fiber to my meals seemed to mitigate the damage of some of my less gut-friendly choices. Or at least it made me feel better about them.

A handful of hemp seeds and a scoop of kimchi on top of gluten-free pasta was a great way to offset the simple carbs. And when vegetables weren't the main event, like when Charlie was in charge of breakfast, I added a spoonful of local kraut from the farmer's market to our plates, which tasted great with homemade harissa turkey sausage and soft scrambled eggs. Overall, edible probiotics were an easy and delicious way to add some health to my hedonism.

The only problem was that despite the fact that the pipes were running smoothly, the more legume-y meals sometimes made me feel like my old friend Violet Beauregarde after she turned into a blueberry.

"There's an old Mexican adage," Justin Sonnenburg relayed, "that the only cure for an intolerance of beans is a steady diet of beans." Gas, he explained, is a natural by-product of all that good fermentation that's happening in your gut. The key is to slowly ramp up your fiber intake so that the bloating doesn't get uncomfortable. Eventually, a big bowl of chili or lentil masala won't affect you the way it used to.

While the qualitative changes were important, it was hard to know what was really going on deep in my intestines without some hard data.

When I finally got my uBiome results back, I felt a little bit like I was finding out my SAT score. And unfortunately, I did just as mediocre on my stool exam, despite there being no math section.

My numbers had increased from the 68th to the 83rd percentile for diversity of species. But my ratios of different phyla hadn't really budged. I found this rather discouraging, since one of the most empowering parts of my gut research was that you can change the course of your gut makeup fairly quickly (within a few weeks).

But perhaps for those of us who have suffered several rounds of mass microbial extinction, getting old populations to take residence again can be an uphill battle—one that just takes time.

The Sweet Spot

The indoor plant experiment—something that I thought would be one of the easier additions of my wellness project—turned out to be a disaster when the hours Charlie spent installing my chic wall garden outnumbered the weeks the plants stayed alive. Whether it was due to the building heat coming on during the first frigid weekend of fall, or the overwatering I might have done to compensate, my succulents soon withered into Donatella Versace shadows of their former selves.

I had better luck with the other living creatures under my care. Becoming a pet owner by proxy was one way to get outside more—especially in the morning—interact with other animals, and feed my microbes at the same time. I was grateful that paying attention to my smallest roommates made me more compassionate toward my two future ones in the process.

When I began investigating the clean-eating side of this challenge, I was hell-bent on finding a perfect probiotic prescription. Unfortunately, as I learned from my gut senseis, there is no such thing as a bacterial silver bullet. Everyone's dose is deeply individual. 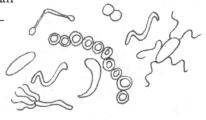 Finding it requires trial and error. And like all supplementation, the efficacy is really only as good as your diet as a whole.

"Destroying your gut bacteria and then trying to replenish them with a probiotic is like draining a full bathtub and replacing the contents with a single cup of water—it's literally a drop in the bucket," wrote Dr. Chutkan.

I would have to keep trying to eat a probiotic a day and resort to taking them in pill form when I was traveling or didn't have access to the kraut jars in my fridge. I was on the right track, even if it would take a while to fill the bucket, and require more than just a little dog hair and kimchi to do so. As my uBiome report confirmed, it would also take patience.

And speaking of patience, I learned that one incentive to stay on the good gut train is what it can do for your mood. Stress is nuanced and mysterious. But there's early evidence that fortifying your gut bacteria can lessen depression, while states of panic can degrade the ecosystem in your gut.

Perhaps my anxiety over Baron the Beagle's hair had done more damage than any bad microbe he might have tracked inside my apartment. My final set of challenges would be to quiet my mind once and for all, and hopefully, the experiments would help me find a better chill pill than what was in my probiotic bottle.

Nurturing your good bacteria is a big part of gut health. But there are also plenty of other processes that happen before your food ever reaches the small intestine. Here are some lifestyle adjustments that can help keep your gut workers happy and your digestive system working like a well-oiled machine.

1. *Try to use antibiotics only when absolutely necessary.* Dr. Chutkan recommended engaging your doctor in a respectful conversation around the following questions: Is the antibiotic treating an actual infection or is it preventative? What's the worst thing that would happen if I didn't take anything? If you decide to go forward with the prescribed meds, increase your probiotic intake throughout the course and for a month afterward to make sure you're replenishing what gets killed. Take your probiotic as far away from the antibiotic as possible (e.g., mid-afternoon if you're taking pills in the morning and at night).

2. *Supplement with bottled bugs.* Eating lacto-fermented foods every day is ideal. But if you're facing an extreme extinction (like during frequent antibiotic courses), get a little help from the supplement aisle. Much like the vitamin industry as a whole, over-the-counter probiotics lack oversight and accountability with the FDA. Products that list the specific strain usually have more data to support their claims, says Ashley Harris, founder of LoveBug Probiotics. For example, *Lactobacillus* (genus) *rhamnosus* (species) GG (strain) was isolated and patented in the 1980s and is the most clinically studied strain in the world. Diversity and count are key, and medical-grade probiotics prescribed by a physician

pack the biggest punch. Regular shoppers should look for something with at least five different strains and a ten-billion-CFU— or colony-forming-unit—count.

3. **Kick the antacids.** Like antibiotics, many over-the-counter pills have unanticipated side effects that can make your gut problems worse in the long run. By reducing your stomach acid with proton pump inhibitors, you create an environment that's more susceptible to foreign invaders. Get out of the habit of popping these pills every time your stomach is upset and grab a bottle of kombucha instead.

4. **Ditch the hand sanitizers and wipes.** Especially during childhood, when the microbiome is being colonized for the years to come, it's important not to wipe out the diversity of species by scrubbing and killing them with chemicals. Regular castile soap and warm water is all you need to protect yourself from the bad guys. Toss all your antibacterial products, including harmful household cleaners, for the sake of your long-term immunity.

5. **Eat the whole plant.** Though all vegetables are great for feeding your bugs, the stringier, woodier varieties, like asparagus, artichokes, leeks, and onions, have a lot of fiber and are also high in inulin, a complex carb favored by gut flora. The tougher parts are gut gold—don't throw them away! Asparagus stems are delicious when pureed (Shrimp and Asparagus Pesto Pasta Salad with Chives, page 308).

6. **Have beans, nuts, and seeds at the ready.** Beans are one of the world's oldest superfoods and were the strongest constant in the diets of every centenarian population studied in Dan Buettner's *The Blue Zones Solution: Eating and Living Like the World's Healthiest People.* Nuts were also the snack of choice. And it's

no surprise that all of these fiber- and complex-carb-rich foods
are favorites of your gut bacteria too. Have some cooked beans,
chopped nuts, and hemp seeds on hand to sprinkle on top of your
soups and salads.

7. ***Add a spoonful of bugs.*** Kefir is great in smoothies or dressings
    (like in my Grilled Romaine Hearts with Roasted Shallots, Arti-
    choke Hearts, and Kefir Green Goddess Dressing on page 305),
    kraut and kimchi can be used to top homemade sausage or grain
    bowls, and organic white miso can be whisked into soups. Be care-
    ful about cooking fermented foods—too much heat will kill the
    bacteria. If adding to hot preparations, make sure to stir in right
    before serving, off the stove.

8. ***Keep a poop log.*** There's often a surprising disconnect for people
    between what goes in their mouth and what comes out the other
    end. Taking the time to record the scoop on your poop, in con-
    junction with a food journal, can give you a wealth of information
    about your body. Ideally, your first bowel movement should hap-
    pen shortly after waking because the liver has been working over-
    night getting rid of yesterday's waste. You want the color to be
    medium brown (think, 60 percent cacao), the weight to be bulky
    and compact, and for there to be a clean wipe.

9. ***Using a stool helps your stool come out quicker.*** Apparently
    our pervasive "sitting diseases" extends to the bathroom sphere as
    well. We'd all be better off pooping as we did in the backcoun-
    try, squatting over an open hole in the ground with no stacks of
    Us Weekly magazines nearby. Luckily, this position can be re-
    created while still using your modern toilet. All you need is a set
    of small stools or a platform to raise your knees. This opens the
    colon and gets your intestines into the proper position for evac-

uation. Though my Squatty Potty looks like something that belongs to a toddler, I've become addicted to it and can never go back.

10. *Use bentonite clay when you're in a bind and need a bind.* Exercising "watchful waiting" can be difficult if you're experiencing a diarrhea emergency on the side of a mountain or in the middle of a work trip. Activated charcoal capsules have always been my go-to for absorbing unwanted toxins before I get heavy-duty meds involved. But clay might be even more effective for critical conditions. Stir a tablespoon into some water or mix together with applesauce. It binds to unwanted contaminants and slows your system down.

11. *Give your gut a break after lunch.* Since your digestive system weakens as the day goes on, it's better to eat raw foods before four p.m. and cooked foods, which are easier to break down, afterward. Try also to eat your bigger meals earlier in the day to make way for lighter dinners, like all those skinny French women do.

12. *Chew your food.* Saliva is such an important piece of our digestive puzzle and we often eat like anacondas, swallowing our food down so fast that our bellies are forced to do most of the work. Take a few extra seconds to actually chew your food—your tummy will thank you!

GRILLED ROMAINE HEARTS WITH ROASTED SHALLOTS, ARTICHOKE HEARTS, AND KEFIR GREEN GODDESS DRESSING

Serves 2 to 4

This recipe is the healthy hedonist alternative to an anemic, blue cheese–bombed iceberg wedge salad. It has a plethora of gut all-stars: fibrous almonds and artichokes, lacto-fermented kefir, and inulin-infused shallots. The charred hearts of romaine make for a beautiful presentation if served to company but also taste great raw if you don't want to bother with a grill.

....

4 medium shallots, peeled and quartered

2 cups quartered artichoke hearts (if frozen, thawed; if canned, rinsed and drained)

2 tablespoons olive oil, plus more for brushing

$^1/_2$ teaspoon sea salt

$^1/_2$ avocado

1 garlic clove

2 tablespoons freshly squeezed lemon juice

$^1/_3$ cup fresh basil leaves, tightly packed

$^1/_3$ cup fresh mint leaves, tightly packed

$^2/_3$ cup lactose-free plain kefir

2 hearts of romaine, washed and halved lengthwise

$^1/_4$ cup roasted almonds, chopped

1. Preheat the oven to 425°F. Line a rimmed baking sheet with parchment paper.

2. Toss the shallots, artichoke hearts, olive oil, and ½ teaspoon salt together on the prepared baking sheet with your hands until well coated. Arrange in an even layer and roast until browned and caramelized, 25 to 35 minutes.

3. Meanwhile, in the bowl of a small food processor, puree the avocado, garlic, lemon juice, basil, mint, and kefir until smooth. Add water by the tablespoon until you obtain a ranch dressing–like consistency. You should have 1½ cups of dressing.

4. Heat an indoor grill pan or cast-iron skillet. Dry the romaine with a kitchen towel and lightly brush the cut sides with olive oil. Grill the lettuce heads cut-side down over high heat until char marks have formed and the leaves begin to wilt, 3 to 5 minutes. Transfer to a serving platter.

5. Top the grilled romaine with the roasted shallots and artichokes, drizzle with ½ cup of the dressing, and garnish with the almonds. Serve immediately with the remaining green goddess dressing on the side.

HEALTHY HEDONIST TIPS

Everything here can be made in advance except for the romaine. If you're packing this as a brown bag lunch, simply cut the lettuce into wedges or chop it for a more office-friendly eating experience. The dressing keeps for up to 2 weeks and is one of the reasons this salad is such a good fit for the follicular phase of your cycle. In addition to being high in fiber, avocados are great for easing the transition to ovulation by promoting progesterone production.

MARKET SWAPS

The beauty of kefir is that many brands are completely lactose-free. If you can't find it, sub ¼ cup full-fat Greek yogurt and ¼ cup water. If you're avoiding dairy, use mayonnaise or Vegenaise (as in traditional green goddess dressings). You're most likely to find jarred artichoke hearts in the Italian specialty section of your market, though some stores do sell frozen versions. If the hearts are whole, simply quarter them by hand.

SHRIMP AND ASPARAGUS PESTO PASTA SALAD WITH CHIVES

Serves 4

You always want to try to use the whole plant when cooking, not just for the sake of your wallet and the environment but because the tough, stringy parts are often the healthiest for your gut! The woody bottom portion of asparagus stalks usually gets escorted out of the house by way of a trash bag. They may not be all that appetizing on their own, but blanched and then pureed? Say hello to your new go-to pesto, friends.

....

1 bunch of asparagus (about 1 pound)

8 ounces gluten-free fusilli

1 cup fresh or frozen peas

$^{1}/_{4}$ cup, plus 1 tablespoon olive oil

$^{3}/_{4}$ pound large shrimp, peeled and deveined

$^{1}/_{2}$ teaspoon sea salt

Freshly ground black pepper

$^{1}/_{2}$ cup coarsely chopped fresh chives, plus more for garnish

2 garlic cloves

3 tablespoons freshly squeezed lemon juice (about 1 lemon)

$^{1}/_{4}$ cup walnut halves

1. Bring a large pot of salted water to a boil and prepare an ice bath. Tie the asparagus together into a bundle with two 10-inch pieces of kitchen twine. Blanch the asparagus until bright green and tender, about 3 minutes. Use tongs to transfer the asparagus to the ice bath. (You can also rinse in a colander under cold water to lock in the color and stop the cooking.)

2. Bring the water back to a boil, add the pasta, and cook according to the package directions. During the last minute of cooking, add the peas. Drain and shake out any excess water. Transfer to a large mixing bowl.

3. Meanwhile, heat 1 tablespoon olive oil in a large cast-iron skillet. Season the shrimp with sea salt and pepper and arrange in an even layer in the pan. Cook until curled and lightly charred on both sides, about 3 minutes total. Add the shrimp to the pasta bowl.

4. Untie the asparagus bunch and cut the stalks into three equal pieces. Transfer the woody bottom thirds to the bowl of a food processor, along with the chives, garlic, lemon juice, walnuts, ½ teaspoon salt, and ¼ cup olive oil. Puree until smooth.

5. Coarsely chop the remaining asparagus and add to the pasta bowl.

6. Pour the pesto over the pasta mixture and toss until well coated. Transfer to a serving bowl and garnish with additional finely chopped chives. Serve warm or at room temperature.

HEALTHY HEDONIST TIPS

Keeping your diet full of fibrous veggies is important on a daily basis, but it's particularly helpful during the ovulatory phase of your menstrual cycle, when your body needs extra help eliminating surplus estrogen. Make sure your gluten-free pasta isn't packed with processed white flours. Stick with quinoa or brown rice as the base—my favorite fusilli brands are Andean Dream and Jovial.

MARKET SWAPS

Any bright green herb will work well in the pesto. Keep it traditional by adding basil or parsley, or give it a hint of anise flavor with fresh tarragon. Scallions can add some of the onion flavor you'd lose by swapping chives. Walnuts are a great affordable option to add a nutty body to the pesto, but if you can find pine nuts on sale, their flavor when toasted is unparalleled. And, of course, you can easily make this pasta vegan by skipping the shrimp.

RELAXATION STATION

LEARNING TO TAKE MY SOUL VITAMINS

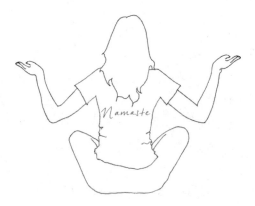

On freeing myself from stress and finding a better way to start the day.

When the subway inexplicably skips my stop or the line at Trader Joe's wraps around the block, as a busy New Yorker I have to take a breath and ask myself, "What would my calm twin do right now?" Even everyday noises—the clatter of the corner bodega opening its storefront, the person eating popcorn with his mouth open at the movie theater, the app notifications I can't ever seem to turn off—can throw my system into fight-or-flight mode, threatening to dismantle my inner calm twin without my even knowing it.

Stress can be extremely corrosive for the body, fueling a variety of the issues I unpacked vis-à-vis this project, including bad skin, dehydration, insomnia, hormone imbalance, damaged gut flora, and acute back pain.

Physical problems are endlessly driven by mental ailments and vice versa. But often it's hard to tell where the first structural screw came loose, upstairs or down.

My body had come a long way since I found myself fighting back tears in the dermatologist's office before starting this project. But during so many of my wellness challenges, it seemed like my mind was the invisible fence holding me back from fully healing. And it was clear that the time I spent zoning out on the couch in front of *The Voice* or with my face planted in the cradle of a massage chair wasn't helping me unwind on a deeper level.

Of all my challenge areas, I had the hardest time deciding which experiments to focus on to de-stress, which, at times, became rather stressful. Because we are complicated emotional beings, relieving the mind of its tormentors is a profoundly individual and complex process. True decompression involves clearing out the cobwebs of bad emotions—the kind that can make you feel like you're riding bitch between Chris Christie and Mama June in even the most relaxing of settings.

I realized that this project was, in some ways, part of the problem. Reconciling all I'd learned from my wellness experiments was creating its own special brand of pressure. There were so many takeaways and best practices, and so little time in my day to make good on all of them.

I wanted to tame my mind, which really meant figuring out how to tame my *life*. I needed to reprioritize, cut back, and say no to the things that caused me more worry than joy, so that fitting de-stressing into my busy day didn't become a burden in and of itself.

Rise and Shine

At the beginning of my project, when I sought out advice from experts in various spheres of the health world, many of the responses to my One Big Question fell under the blanket category of "small acts of self-tithing." As

Acu Heidi put it, "We spend so much time renting out mental space to other people's problems, spending ten percent of your day on yourself is like taking your soul vitamins."

I wondered what would happen if I made quality alone time a mandatory part of my every day—an activity to ward off stress instead of something I defaulted to only during certain parts of my cycle or when my nerves had already been fried by one too many choruses of "Shout." I needed a consistent system for shifting my mind from chaos to calm—for making my mornings just about me.

One thing I'd learned the hard way over the course of my project—through my sleep, my eating, and even my bowels—is that there's nothing the body loves more than a reliable timetable. The mind is no different. Routine is an essential part of forming habits. It hardwires the brain for success, and it takes some of the unhealthy stress of decision making off the table.

Over the course of my project, my morning habits had changed considerably from the pants-less email-writing and coffee-chugging days of my past. My sleep experiments made me recommit to a firm wake-up time, and turning my cell phone on airplane mode before climbing into bed meant I was less likely to be mindlessly deleting Gilt emails each morning before my feet even hit the ground. During back health month, I started setting aside the fifteen minutes while my green tea steeped for my pelvic-floor exercises. Since the vice detox and throughout my clean-eating months, I'd been whipping up a quick breakfast to keep up with my high-fiber, low-sugar protocol—the best way to start the day for all of my organs. And thanks to my new temperature charting practice, the first thing I now grabbed for in bed was my thermometer instead of my phone.

There wasn't enough time for all of these prework practices, though, and rarely was I able to be consistent from day to day. For my final set of experiments, I wanted to take a step away from all of these tactics for my body and try two new ones for my mind: journaling and what most people agree is the most important element of anyone's mind routine, that panacea of stress—meditation.

By the end, I could look back on my year's worth of rituals, put all the pieces together, and decide on the best use of my precious morning "me time" going forward.

The Sound of Silence

Over the years, I had made stabs at meditating, with mixed results. I had tried apps. I had tried Deepak. I had tried a weird hypnosis exercise that involved visualizing my first pet, a guinea pig named Piglet. None of them gave me the mental tools I needed to wrestle my brain to the ground during times of deep anxiety.

Of all of my wellness expenditures, getting a formal meditation training would be the biggest investment—a luxury when compared to the thirteen dollars a month I might otherwise spend on a Headspace subscription. I knew if I was serious about starting a practice, though, I would need some structure, hand-holding, and an in-person teacher to guide me. The four-day program, paid off monthly, would amount to a yearlong gym membership for my mind. But I hoped that if I stuck with it, meditation would be a skill that would pay dividends in every area of my life for the years to come.

The power to increase reaction time has made athletes like Kobe Bryant and Derek Jeter look to meditation to improve their performance. Artists see it as a boon to their creativity. Career-driven start-up entrepreneurs rave about their newfound focus and productivity. And other regular Joes and Janes just notice how all of their relationships seem to fall into place when they are more grounded in the present and not sending passive-aggressive text messages all the time.

Even the insurance company Blue Cross Blue Shield discovered that meditators were cheaper to cover. Their data, which followed subjects for five years, found that those who practiced had 50 percent fewer hospital admissions compared to non-meditators and controls. There were also fewer instances of cancer, heart attacks, and even car crashes.

These were the types of fun facts that Ben Turshen rattled off during the first hour of his introductory talk on the power of meditation.

"Under normal circumstances, our brain is like an orchestra during warm-up—it's just a bunch of noise," explained my new guru. "But meditating is like waving the conductor's baton; it brings the whole performance together."

The studio was a sparsely decorated corner office in midtown Manhattan. A table in the back offered tea and snacks, along with printed paraphernalia like Ben's signature "Do not disturb, I'm meditating" doorknob hangers. As I reclined into one of the hard-backed floor cushions—chicer versions of the Crazy Creek chairs you'd find around a campfire—he told the group of prospective meditators about his background as an anxious child turned anxious corporate attorney. Ready for a new approach after years of taking Ambien to sleep, Adderall to wake up, and Xanax to stay relaxed, Ben found himself at a Buddhist meditation center. Only, his time spent in a stiff pretzel position on the floor, desperately trying to push thoughts from his head, left him feeling more tortured. Finally, he found Vedic meditation, a practice that seemed to better appreciate his monkey mind.

"Vedic means 'from the Vedas,' which are an ancient Indian body of knowledge," Ben said, as a dozen adults of all ages listened attentively, hands fighting the urge to take notes on their phones. "They were an oral tradition, passed down through generations of pandits. But the practice still applies to modern life because it's designed for the householder, not the monk."

This was reassuring, as was the fact that my new guru was wearing skinny jeans and a plaid button-down instead of prayer beads and an orange robe.

Ben reminded us that the mind is a constant flight risk. When left to its own devices, it fixates on the past or, worse, speculates on the future, both of which can cause suffering. In many ways, though, the mind itself is predictable—it has the emotional maturity of a toddler and is constantly looking for where it'll get the most unadulterated pleasure.

Vedic meditation uses this tendency to its advantage.

"There's no point in battling your mind's cravings, hence why I've provided plenty of snacks and blankets for all those who feel called toward warmth or hunger," Ben told us with a booming chuckle. "And this is also where your mantra comes in."

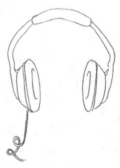

The mantra creates a pleasant diversion, as if leading the mind away from suffering with a trail of berry-flavored fruit snacks. It isn't necessarily the most beautiful-sounding word, just as the most dynamic guy at a cocktail party might not be the most pleasant to be around—they are designed to be fascinating. A mantra is like your mind's very own Justin Bieber: you can't help but be drawn to it.

After we'd each received our mantra privately and had our first meditation, Ben outlined the nuts and bolts of the Vedic practice:

1. *Twenty minutes, twice a day.* As Ben acknowledged, no one decides to sign up for meditation class because they have an extra forty minutes in their day. But the Transcendental and Vedic sets are married to this time breakdown as the optimal dose. It's the mind's equivalent of a three-for-two deal. While one meditation resonates in the body as one session, fortifying your practice with a second meditation has the impact of three sessions.

2. Don't eat or caffeinate beforehand. The best time for meditation is first thing in the morning before food or drink. When your body's digesting, it's dedicating energy to that task. This works against you as a meditator, when you're trying to get your body to rest. You're asking it to do two opposing things at once.

3. Don't meditate too close to bedtime. Meditation isn't an end in and of itself. You want to feel the benefits—the focus, creativity, and increase in performance—out in the world. Going straight to bed defeats that purpose. Also, once your body has experienced such a deep state of rest (said to be at least twice as intense as your best sleep), it will probably be too energized and alert to doze off easily. Because of this, the optimal time for your second session is mid-afternoon, sometime after lunch and before dinner.

4. Support your back, not your head. Meditating doesn't have to be painful. Sitting cross-legged on a hard stone floor with your hip crying out for mercy is not a necessary mind-body test. The Vedic householder technique is all about being comfortable. Choose any position that fits the bill as long as your head isn't supported; otherwise, you will end up sleeping instead of meditating.

5. Self-monitor. You don't want to undo all that good relaxation you just fostered with a loud alarm. It's better to come out on your own. Your body will begin to get a little active after about twenty minutes. If it makes you less anxious about getting out the door to a meeting on time, set an emergency timer for twenty-five minutes and choose something soothing like crickets on a low volume.

6. Take the time to settle. It's most productive to ease out of your meditation period, taking at least two minutes at the end to slowly come out of the session. Even if you only have time for a shorter session, devote at least two minutes for that readjustment period.

Background Noise

After my prior lack of success with guided meditations and apps, I expected there to be a learning curve. But halfway into my first group meditation, I was feeling a light hallucinogenic buzz. My fingers, intertwined in my lap, became one gently vibrating glob. As I walked home, I felt a mental calm and physical high. Colors were somehow brighter. The steam coming out of a manhole, that much trippier. And as I meandered through Whole Foods, not even the Chelsea mothers blocking the aisles with their strollers could get me down.

Perhaps my newfound patience was, in part, a product of exhaustion. Ben warned that it's normal to feel some fatigue when you first start meditating—a natural by-product of your body shedding all the tension it has been holding on to for decades. Like working out, some people get hit immediately by this initial "soreness," and for others it takes a few days to kick in. True to my experiences with physical exercise, that night I fell into bed like a helpless stuffed animal.

The next morning, I waited impatiently as Charlie took his shower and got ready for work, already conscious of how my new routine was cutting into the workday. At 8:32 a.m. I sat down on the couch to begin. Just as I started finding the mantra, it seemed that the only thing occupying my head was the sound of sirens outside. I tried to concentrate, but there was no way to mentally muscle through it. After a few minutes, I peeked through the blinds to see people standing aghast as firefighters stormed the building next door. I heard the key in the lock. Charlie had come back to make sure I was in a fully conscious state should

I have to evacuate. (Clearly, he thought I was already a much better meditator than I was.)

I relayed this story during class that evening as we went around the
room sharing our first solo experiences. My peers nodded in agreement.
For me it was sirens; for others, it was the annoying sound of the radiator,
car horns, or attention-hungry children.

"Every time I sit down to meditate, my leg starts itching uncontrol-
lably," a svelte redhead in a Theory pantsuit reported. "It's like I'm allergic
to relaxation."

Ben told us to mentally note these disturbances. It's a lot easier to
bounce back to a place of calm after scratching your leg than spending
twenty minutes trying not to scratch your leg. Pretending these distractions didn't exist wouldn't do us any favors. Also, in my case, doing so
might have resulted in burning to a crisp.

During that night's session, I tried to remember his guidance. Ham-
mering the mantra into your brain like a nail, tying it to the rhythm
of the breath, or tirelessly reciting it won't allow
you to fully drop into your meditation. Keep that
spiritual gibberish in a choke hold for twenty
minutes, and you'll emerge with TMJ and not a
whole lot of transcendence to show for your
efforts.

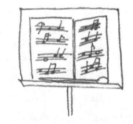

My mind did wander, but eventually it entered a sort of trance. There
was some activity, but it felt dreamlike; I was partially removed from it.
Everything in my head became fainter. The orchestra had started playing, and I was lost in the harmonies.

Brain Drain

After a month of meditating every morning, I felt like the practice was cemented enough that I was ready to add a new layer to my morning routine: journaling.

I'd always kept notebooks but never developed a strong habit of daily writing. My leather Moleskines were there to capture the kernel of an idea, random notes on my wellness experiments, some reflections during introspective menstrual moments, or therapeutic rants about various micro-aggressions toward Charlie, clients, or other confidants. As a writer, it felt frivolous throwing away my finite reservoir of words on something I couldn't use toward my daily (paying) assignments. And if I tried to make my morning journaling a productive part of my workday, wouldn't that turn my "me time" into yet another chore?

Others didn't seem to share this outlook. Many of the self-employed superstars I knew swore by writing "morning pages," a concept that Julia Cameron, the prolific writer and nursemaid to blocked creatives everywhere, introduced in her best-selling book *The Artist's Way: A Spiritual Path to Higher Creativity*.

Before reading it, I thought I understood the general concept: putting pen to paper first thing in the morning has a sort of magical quality. It's the time when our subconscious is at its most permeable. Dreams are easier to pluck from the depths. Thoughts are at their purest. And doing a "brain drain" is more apt to lead to an unexpected clue or stroke of genius.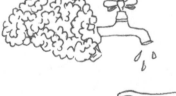

When I finally picked up *The Artist's Way*, though, I realized I had partially missed the point.

One of the cardinal rules of morning pages is that you don't reread your words. If meditation is a way to close the door to the mental attic for twenty minutes, then the pages' purpose is to clear out all of the junk in one stream of consciousness. It's not an exercise for creative mastery or inspiration. First and foremost, morning pages are there to help you get out of your own way.

"These daily morning meanderings are not meant to be *art*. Or even *writing*," Cameron says. "Although occasionally colorful, the morning pages are often negative, frequently fragmented, often self-pitying, repetitive, stilted or babyish, angry or bland—even silly-sounding."

If so, you're on the right track, she explains. Because this is the stuff that's holding you back, and not just from your creativity. These are the worries and petty cares that stand between you and a happy life.

"It is difficult to complain about a situation morning after morning, month after month, without being moved to constructive action. The pages lead us out of despair into undreamed-of solutions."

Meditation puts negative thinking on hold. Morning pages beat it out of the mind like a dusty pillow. They put a mirror into your hands and force you to look deep within for the answers.

For me, this might have been the last frontier of healing.

Written in the Stars

If there was ever a time in my life that I needed a brain drain, it was now.

As I turned the final corner of my project, I was getting closer to another deadline: the big 3-0.

I didn't expect to have a Jessie Spano–style meltdown, but as the days crept closer and closer to my birthday, I felt the weight of one door closing—in this case, a decade—and the next one opening. I didn't need my life to be settled in the traditional sense by way of a husband or a mortgage. (Though I had hoped to own a real dining-room table by now.) It was more that I'd expected to emerge from the dark tunnel of uncertainty that haunted most of my twenties. That the gnawing sense of unknowing would evaporate like the morning mist and I would wake up at thirty having my shit together.

As the weeks drew nearer, that didn't seem likely to happen. My mornings may have been more under control, but I wasn't sure that journaling and meditating alone could remedy the fact that my plate had been overfilled with questions at the emotional buffet. I was feeling restless in New York. So many of my wellness challenges made me realize how much healthier my life would be with more space, sunshine, and yoga pants. Less black, more balance. But the dominoes were not mine alone to arrange.

Thanks to the new decade on the horizon, my short-term questions about what city I should live in and whether I'd be able to make a living there were compounded by the bigger unknowns. Was this the man I was supposed to spend the rest of my life with? What would happen if our visions for the next chapter diverged? In a relationship, when does compromise turn into an unhealthy sacrifice? And how can you tell when it's really fear that's steering you in one direction or another?

In order to let go of the anxiety of not knowing what my life would look like on paper after my project was complete, to paper—to the pages—I turned.

As my mother once told me, the process of writing is really the process of being alone in the world—lost in the desert with nothing but your thoughts. Like pigeon pose in yoga, it's best to just breathe through the discomfort.

As I leaned into this uncertainty through my journal, I could feel my mind coming back into orbit.

For all the lingering shame I felt in expressing some of my uglier feelings honestly on paper, I also experienced an unexpected streak of empathy. To balance the dirty spirals of my mental crap, I tried to end each session by writing down three things I was grateful for.

Several studies have shown that gratitude has a stronger link to health than any other emotion. So on days when my mind was feeling its least healthy, I got all that torment down on paper and then attempted to find the antidote in a few short lines.

When I was at a loss for brain dump topics, I wrote letters I would never send. To Baron the Beagle, for accepting me despite my reluctance to open my whole home and heart to him. Many letters to Charlie for being so tolerant of my faults—especially my tendency to unfurl Egyptian scrolls' worth of his—and for forcing me to embrace the full package of his love, when fear sometimes made me want to return it to sender.

Even my thyroid—that sweet, sad sponge below my throat—was worthy of a morning page love letter. As I reflected on my wellness project, a deep admiration for my body and its many capabilities emerged. And as I reached the finish line, that awe turned even further inward.

Above all, my "me time" allowed me to redirect some much-needed compassion toward myself. I had to push through a lot of inner doubt, outer weaknesses, and pervasive pad Thai cravings to get to this point. And teetering at the edge of a new decade, ready to turn the page, I was incredibly proud of myself and grateful for the journey.

Perhaps you can't tell the difference between fear and courage until you reach the other side.

The Sweet Spot

With the addition of morning pages to my routine, I was forced to confront the first leg of "putting it all together."

On the one hand, I liked doing my meditation session immediately so that I could sip my tea and eat while writing, but I found that my pages flowed better when I did them first thing. I had an easier time remembering my dreams, and the more I wrote about them, the more my subconscious seemed to offer up the subsequent night.

I posed the order question to Julia Cameron on Twitter and she agreed: "Morning pages to skim any crap off the top and allow for a beautiful meditation."

Well, then.

On mornings when I was away from home or didn't have time for twenty minutes of each prong, I allowed myself a micro-routine that took less than ten minutes: just five minutes of quiet with my eyes closed, and a few lines of gratitude. I also started adding in something quick to get my blood flowing and energize my body for the day: five sun salutations, jumping jacks, or leg lifts in supported bridge pose.

I made more of an effort to prepare a breakfast option during my batch-cooking sessions so that I didn't have to worry about it in the morning and could just tee up a jar of chia pudding or overnight oats to enjoy alongside my tea when I finally sat down at the computer.

Trying to squeeze in too many activities threatened to defeat the purpose of my pursuit. Having that time to myself in the morning was a luxury. It allowed me to get quiet, set my own pace, and ease into the day before my inbox opened and swallowed me whole.

After my setback with the parasite, it felt good to have a system of surrender.

I wanted to reach the end of my year of experiments having solved all of my problems. But I learned the hard way that there was only so much I could control, throughout this project and beyond. The most important thing was that I now had a new arsenal of tools in my back pocket. And meditation was that missing piece for my monkey mind.

On busy afternoons, even when I failed to log a formal session, it was helpful to know that if I felt anxious or impatient or unfocused, I could always close my eyes for five minutes to reset. These quick doses didn't necessarily cue the orchestra. But they quickly retuned my thoughts to the proper key.

A little over a month after the class ended, I began to lose my meditation mojo. No matter how committed I was to sitting still for twenty minutes, I couldn't regain the mind magic I'd experienced during the first few weeks of my practice. Instead of effortlessly bringing my thoughts back to the mantra, the mundane worries would take over.

Was it beginner's luck? A loss of novelty? Or was I just better able to ground myself in my meditation when surrounded by ten other humans emanating the same blissed-out energy?

One of the benefits of investing in a formal training—the lifelong gym membership for my mind—was that I could always rely on the power of my teacher and fellow meditators to ground me.

The trick, perhaps, was to develop a habit of mindfulness. I realized that in my diligence to craft a set morning routine, I had lost some of the intentions behind my practices. Meditation had become just another thing I had to do. And because I wasn't always thoughtful about its purpose and clear about my intentions when I sat down to do it, the end result lost some of its luster.

In class, it was clear what we were there for. Not just *what* we'd be doing but *why* we were doing it. Perhaps talking about the benefits of meditation before we began made them stronger.

To get my groove back at home, I tried lighting a candle at the beginning and blowing it out at the end of my session to create firmer context and to remember my goal of focus and relaxation before I started.

But if I had a day when my mantra got defeated by the "is this even working?" train of thought, I tried to be kinder to myself and remember that twenty minutes of stillness was a gift. Even when the distractions got to me, noting them was still grounding. They were happening in the present moment, not ten miles in the future.

My mind wasn't being thrown into the outer atmospheres like a boomerang.

1. *Create a micro-morning routine.* There are always days when, despite all our well-groomed habits, we are more harried than usual. Rather than skip your morning ritual, do an abbreviated version. For me, that was five minutes of meditation, writing down three things I was grateful for, and doing five sun salutations or pelvic-floor exercises.

2. *Practice everyday mindfulness.* Apps like Headspace are great for grounding you on the go. You can use them to tune in to your mind and tune out the subway or the office. Or, you can simply choose one activity and focus on being present. Brushing your teeth, showering, getting the mail . . . anything. Instead of thinking of dishwashing as a chore, I now try to use it as an opportunity to push other thoughts from my head and, instead, focus on the water, the soap, and the feeling of getting crusted quinoa off a pot left in the sink.

3. *Create affirmations.* These written intentions allow you to imbue the day with the power of wishful thinking. If you're a planner like me, simply take five minutes at the beginning of the week and think about what you'd most like to accomplish. Write down your goals in purposeful language and read them to yourself every morning. For example: "I will finish my chapter on stress by the end of the week, and the process will be joyous, not stressful." You

can also focus on a more long-term goal, or simply read an inspiring quote to remind you of your purpose.

4. *Wear a complaint bracelet.* When my friend Sarah went through a dark period, her mother gave her a red bracelet to snap her out of her own negativity. Every time Sarah complained, she had to switch the bracelet to the other wrist. A fitness tracker band can work well for this. Include harmful self-talk or internal monologues of doubt as reasons for switching. It's a good physical reminder to pop your balloon of pessimism before it has a chance to slowly suffocate your spirit.

5. *Perform a random act of kindness.* Perhaps because it's a sister quality to gratitude, generosity is strongly associated with better mental health and longevity. In fact, volunteering has a bigger positive impact on well-being than exercise. Studies on financial happiness find that people who give some of their money away are much happier than those who spend it all on themselves. The amount you give is not proportional to the emotional return. You can make small acts of kindness a part of your every day. Leave a love note in a public place. Pay a stranger a compliment. Do your boyfriend's laundry for him when he's out of boxers.

6. *Care for something.* Like other acts of generosity, taking care of another living thing can be centering and rewarding and give you a sense of purpose. This applies to pets, of course. But it can even be accomplished with something as simple as a flower. In one study, nursing home patients who were given the responsibility of caring for a plant had a much lower mortality rate. Plants are also great for your microbiome, so long as you manage to keep it alive.

7. *Turn off phone notifications.* The constant stimulation of our modern world puts more stress on us than we comprehend. But on a more tangible level, we all know the feeling we get when our phone is buzzing or beeping off the hook with demands from others. Switch your email settings to fetch manually, turn off social media notifications, stop checking your feeds every five minutes, and designate some time in the morning and evening for leaving your phone on airplane mode.

8. *Cook comfort food.* Despite all of my wellness experiments, my own answer to the One Big Question remains the same: home-cooked food can give you the emotional and physical fuel you need to live a healthier, happier life. It allows you to put your own definition of nourishment in a bowl to share with others and, more important, to give to yourself. For me, that soul gasoline involves soup and noodles, and especially, noodles in soup.

VIETNAMESE CHICKEN SOUP FOR THE SOUL

Serves 4

In Vietnam, rice noodle soup is traditionally sipped (well, slurped) in the morning. And though I don't believe its place in traditional cuisine is only as a hangover cure, the gelatin and amino acids from the bone broth certainly help you get rehydrated and back on your feet. This "Pho Ga" broth is usually ladled over a mess of noodles and shredded chicken and served alongside a plate of garnishes, including fresh herbs, scallions, onions, and chilies. I love adding sliced bok choy so my body gets just as much from this comforting bowl as my soul does.

....

2½ quarts (10 cups) "Pho Real" Slow Cooker Ginger-Chicken Bone Broth
   (page 162)

8 ounces thin flat brown rice noodles or gluten-free ramen

2 cups shredded cooked chicken (preferably dark meat)

1 large shallot or ½ small yellow onion, thinly sliced

2 heads of baby bok choy, thinly sliced

¼ cup fish sauce

2 tablespoons freshly squeezed lime juice

½ cup fresh basil leaves, coarsely torn

½ cup fresh cilantro leaves

1 serrano chili, thinly sliced

1 lime, cut into wedges

1. In a large stockpot, bring the chicken broth to a simmer. Add the rice noodles and cook according to package directions (about 2 to 3 minutes, usually). Remove from the heat and stir in the chicken, shallot, bok choy, fish sauce, and lime juice.

2. Divide the soup among four bowls and serve alongside the basil, cilantro, chili, and lime wedges.

HEALTHY HEDONIST TIPS

It's fairly easy to find brown rice noodles these days in the Asian food aisle. You can always swap gluten-free linguine, or simply use plain white pad Thai noodles. Lotus Foods makes amazing black rice and millet ramen that work well in this recipe.

MARKET SWAPS

If you made your ginger chicken broth in advance and don't have the leftover meat, simply use a shredded rotisserie chicken. Another option is to sear chicken thighs and simmer them in the broth for 20 minutes until tender, then shred or chop. Add one 15-ounce can of coconut milk and a lemongrass stalk for a creamy version that resembles the Thai soup tom kha gai.

ALMOND-SESAME SOBA ZOODLES WITH QUICK PICKLED VEGGIES

Serves 2 as a main course or 4 as a side

If cold sesame or peanut noodles are part of your usual comfort food rotation, this dish is a great take-out fake-out. Soba noodles are traditionally made from buckwheat, which, contrary to its name, is a gluten-free flour that's rich in protein and fiber. It also has a wonderful earthy flavor that pairs well with toasted sesame oil, creamy almond butter, and bright pickled vegetables from the farmer's market. To make this noodle dish even more veg-centric, I go halvsies with spiralized zucchini. Depending on your preferences, you can, of course, use all soba or all zoodles (see Market Swap notes). But I think this version gives you the best of both worlds.

....

8 ounces buckwheat soba noodles

1 bunch of radishes (about 6 medium), cut into ¹/₂-inch cubes

1 pound cucumber, cut into ¹/₂-inch cubes

¹/₄ cup rice vinegar

2 teaspoons sea salt, divided

¹/₂ cup unsalted almond butter

1 small garlic clove

¹/₄ cup freshly squeezed lime juice (from 2 limes)

2 tablespoons gluten-free tamari

2 teaspoons raw honey

2 teaspoons dark toasted sesame oil

2 large zucchini (about 1 pound), spiralized into thin noodles

1 tablespoon black sesame seeds, for garnish

1. Bring a large pot of salted water to a boil. Cook the soba noodles according to package directions until al dente. Drain and rinse with cool water until room temperature, shaking out all the excess. Transfer to a large mixing bowl and set aside.

2. While the noodles are cooking, in a medium mixing bowl, combine the radishes, cucumber, vinegar, and 1 teaspoon salt. Allow the veggies to marinate for 10 minutes, tossing occasionally.

3. In the bowl of a small food processor, puree the almond butter, garlic, lime juice, tamari, honey, sesame oil, 1 teaspoon salt, and ¼ cup water. Add more water, 1 tablespoon at a time, until you reach the consistency of peanut sauce. Transfer to the mixing bowl with the soba noodles. Add the zucchini and toss until everything is well coated. Divide among serving bowls, top with the quick pickled veggies, and garnish with the sesame seeds.

4. Serve room temperature or cold, alongside your favorite Asian hot sauce.

HEALTHY HEDONIST TIPS

Make sure to look for noodles that are 100 percent buckwheat, as many traditional soba brands now use wheat flour to create sturdier strands. Eden Foods and King Soba are my favorites. Reserve your radish leaves and use them to make a peppery puree. They're a great addition to my asparagus stalk pesto (page 308).

MARKET SWAPS

If you don't own a spiralizer, you can easily just use all packaged noodles. Simply double the quantity of soba and omit the zucchini. Or for a Paleo version, vice versa. Use whatever veggies you find at the market for the quick-pickled topping. Carrots, fennel, or sugar snap peas would work well. To make a Thai version of this dish, swap vermicelli or flat rice noodles for the soba. Omit the sesame oil completely, and sub 2 tablespoons fish sauce for the tamari. Garnish with chopped peanuts instead of sesame seeds.

EPILOGUE

CONNECTING THE DOTS

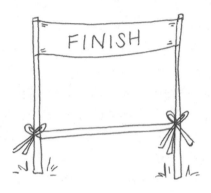

On putting it all together.

Real, lasting change often happens so gradually that it's barely perceptible.

Pain and exhaustion had become my new normal during the worst throes of my autoimmune disease, without my even realizing it. So when the project was over, it took me a few months to fully comprehend how far I'd come.

With the help of many monitoring and tracking devices, rule following and rule breaking, I relearned how to tune in to my body again. Now that it was all over, I tried to take a step back, block out the outside noise—be it a friend, doctor, or sleep monitor—and focus just on how I felt.

And as best practices came and went, and my routines became habitual, I realized that overall, I felt pretty *well*.

From where I stand today, I've gained back much of the vitality I'd lost. Mornings no longer feel like a battle of me versus the bed, and my days aren't a walking continuation of that slumber. Even without doing pelvic-floor exercises on a daily basis, my back has remained spasm-free since the spine experiments. And for the first time since I was diagnosed with Hashimoto's, my blood work doesn't hover on the precipice of numerical disaster. My B_{12}, vitamin D, and other nutrient levels no longer characterize me as a malnourished chef. And I achieved those results without popping hundreds of dollars' worth of supplements. After years of hormonal birth control and courses of antibiotics for my skin, the only medication I take on a regular basis is my thyroid pill and the occasional probiotic. And without all those day-of-the-week pill cases to lug around, taking care of my body feels a lot less like a full-time job.

In terms of external signs, I haven't had a single flare-up of perioral dermatitis since my vice detox. My most glaring, outward-facing symptom of inner chaos has disappeared entirely. And as someone who started from a place of health overwhelm, it was heartening to prove my hypothesis: that twelve months of small baby steps could amount to a big leap forward in my wellness.

It's hard to know which lifestyle changes moved the needle most, even though I took on my health challenges in isolation to better tease out specific results. As someone with an autoimmune disease, I figured it would be apparent which practices packed the biggest punch. What I learned instead is that as a highly sensitive being, *everything* matters. Every toxin, every ounce of stress—it all adds up. And healing any part of the body inevitably takes time.

It took some extremes to end up in a place of moderation. I don't think I could have seen such lasting results without going off the pill, ending the vicious cycle of antibiotics for my acne, or getting rid of a parasite. The same goes for taking some hard lines with my vices and diet, and embracing help from fitness cults to make me strong again. Thanks to those experiments, I finally understand what a perfect health day looks like, even if I don't always have one.

Because I also know that seeking perfection sometimes causes more stress than the end result is worth. The progress I saw at the end of my year confirmed that I can pick and choose my own toxic adventure and the healthy practices that counteract it from day to day. I don't have to do all of the above all at once.

And even if I managed to do so, without a healthy mind, all that hard work would mean nothing.

As I connected the dots of my health, I realized how the internal dialogue of doubt I always thought just made me human—the self-deprecation I had mistaken for modesty—was actually

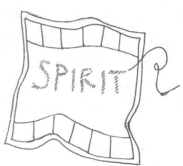

causing me the most harm. Discovering that underlying anxiety was behind my back problems, my insomnia, my adrenal fatigue, and perhaps my autoimmune disease itself was a big revelation that came up again and again during my project. And it was something I didn't fully understand until the end.

My world did not implode when I turned thirty, but the new decade immediately laid out a welcome mat to escort me past the threshold of a new kind of adulthood.

Two weeks before the official project deadline, as I paused and reflected on my year of health ups and downs, Charlie's father passed away. His illness had been on our radar, but the end was quick and heart-wrenching.

In many ways I took on all of these challenges as a framework for coping when the wellness deck was stacked against me. So that when shit did hit the fan, I wouldn't fly into the blades with it. I couldn't help but wonder if this timing was a test from the universe to see if all my new health habits would hold their ground as so many emotional tectonic plates shifted and tremored around me. I wanted to soar across the finish line looking and feeling like I had all my issues under control. But life will always throw you curveballs, and I knew it was up to me to find a more graceful way to shoulder the bumps and bruises.

Thanks to all of the self-knowledge I'd built over the course of my year of wellness, after the initial unraveling of grief, I knew exactly what tools I needed to stitch myself back together. I took Epsom salt baths and meditated. I went for walks to quiet my mind and wrote in my gratitude journal when I couldn't. I cried in Acu Heidi's office, letting her wisdom and needles pull me back to center. And I made bowls of Vietnamese Chicken Soup for the Soul for Charlie, to do whatever bowls of chicken soup are supposed to do.

There's nothing like death to put your own health into perspective. For me, it didn't just make me want to commit even harder to all of my new disease-fighting practices, fortifying my body for the long haul. More so, I felt that Charlie Senior's passing was an even bigger reminder about the importance of healthy hedonism—of savoring every day and filling it with some form of pleasure.

As Ferris Bueller, my hero of hedonism, knew well: life moves pretty fast.

I didn't want to miss it.

I ALSO THOUGHT even further about the pleasures I had given up in the name of my health.

If I looked back on my life, would I really be sad that I didn't eat many months' worth of French macarons? That I left a friend's birthday party early or missed it altogether? Would I feel better about spending an extra hour at my desk writing emails instead of stepping outside to stop and look around?

When the fear of missing out came up, I noticed the parts of my personality that I needed to fight. I had spent my twenties resisting, trying to prove I could transcend my body's limitations with a pitcher of margaritas. That I could still go with the flow, have fun, and be the Cool Girl despite my disease. As I moved through this project, though, and got older in wellness dog years, I learned that the important parts of my world didn't change when I set healthy boundaries.

When I decided to embrace being difficult and stop apologizing, I realized that no apologies were necessary. Friends forgave, hosts adjusted their menus.

The times I did give in to an indulgence, it wasn't necessarily just the reward I was after. Not the strings of melted cheese that danced off a warm quesadilla or the buttery hazelnut filling that oozed out of a light-as-air almond cookie as I took my first bite. More important than what the treat itself brought to my life was what abstaining took away. I needed the freedom to make my own choices in the moment. Because even when we know how to decipher the good from the bad, life is often much sweeter when we occasionally take a bite out of the bad anyway.

Intuition is a muscle. And it's one that my wellness project proved much more valuable to build than my pelvic floor or droopy delts.

Though most of my challenges sought to heal my body, the most striking changes were to my mindset, to honing the lifelong skills I would need to keep my body on track and that *active process* of wellness chugging in the right direction on any given day.

When you have that baseline of body literacy—the ability to tap into what feels right and what doesn't—it can save you a lot of pain down the line. From fad diets and cult workouts. From expert listicles and well-meaning but misguided physicians. And from all the time, money, and energy that those things cost.

My journey would have faced many dead ends and downslides if it weren't for the pieces of advice I received from the capable team I built around me, but how to apply them was up to me and me alone.

AN IMPORTANT FOOTNOTE in my healing came a month after my project ended, when I left the space that contained so many sick memories behind.

With all of the shake-ups in his corner, it became clear that my need for change would have to be satisfied in the near vicinity and, for Charlie's sake, not involve moving three thousand miles away. So at the end of February, after four long years, I bid farewell to my sleeping loft and moved my belongings to a new Brooklyn apartment with large windows (and no LED signs outside), ample counter space, and, unlike my previous home, doors.

It took a few months after the thirty mark, but thanks to the furniture I inherited from my other half, I did finally get that dining-room table.

Charlie and I quickly discovered during the packing process that you plus me equals a lot of stuff. So we both spent the first part of the cohabitation process getting rid of a lot of it. As I invoked the cutthroat criteria of Marie Kondo and deposited wellness doodads in donation bags, it became clear how so many of the objects I had bought to heal my body didn't bring me joy (or much healing).

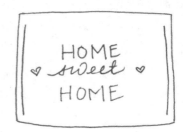

The process of packing my life into boxes was in many ways its own year in review. Not just of my project, but of the half decade before it when I was desperately grabbing at straws. Out went the magnetic back brace, the earthing mat, the foam wedge, the orange blue light–blocking glasses. And though it had brought me some joy, it was time for me to thank the Richard Simmons DVD and find it a new home.

From the back shelves of my kitchen cabinets I purged many long-forgotten superfoods and, from my bathroom, some lasting vestiges of my chemical past—and even some unnecessary naturals I'd hoarded in my green present.

Finally, I faced the one part of my cabinet I hadn't purged during my project: the medicine trays, where years of pills, tinctures, and powders had been accumulating. Like the contents of my other cabinets, I had convinced myself that one day I might need these things. But unlike the others, holding on to them was like waiting for the other shoe to drop: for the day when my body would crash again and the only thing holding me up would be a sack of supplements.

I pulled out the various bottles, not even remembering what half of them were for, until I got to the three Gloria the Healer had given me. I remembered my feelings of relief and gratitude as I held them for the first time. Then the pain and anger I felt when I realized they were doing more harm than good. And *then* the shame and frustration when it hit me that I had put so much hope into the promise of a pill.

I dumped them in the trash where they belonged.

NOT EVERYONE CAN CHANGE their circumstances by picking up and moving, and shedding dead weight and blocked energy in the process. But I didn't need to go far to experience a perspective shift. All it took was a small change in scenery.

Once we were all under the same roof, my attitude toward being a canine stepmother changed. As my project-ambassador-from-afar Gretchen Rubin says, "If you can't get out of it, get into it." And that's exactly what I did.

Besides creating some
healthy literal boundaries
within the space, I began
a new experiment: the
Wellness Project, Doggy
Edition. Between the
changes in diet, and Baron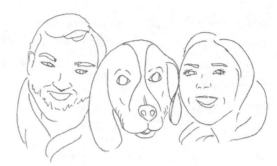
the Beagle's new wogging regimen (a daily thirty minutes outside with
me), he lost seven pounds. His ample hair gets brushed and sprayed with a
homemade mixture of natural oils daily. And even though I'm not going
to divest my stock in Swiffer anytime soon, these changes allow me to
experience a serotonin and oxytocin rush when a wet black nose greets me
first thing as part of my new morning routine.

As for my other roommate, I had spent a lot of my year nagging Charlie
about his own health practices, giving him seminars on the world's many
toxic dangers and stressing out about the advice he didn't heed. I would
sometimes notice his eyes glaze over (and/or roll back) at dinner when I
launched into fun facts about the chlorine in tap water, the ractopamine in
pork, and the cervical fluid in my drawers.

I realized halfway through the year that I was doing a disservice to
the purpose of my project with these diatribes. I wanted to help people
find the balance between health and hedonism, not to become slaves to
their bodies, and certainly not to live in fear. While I sought to teach
others everything I'd learned, I had to try to do so in a way that didn't
impose any sense of right and wrong on them.

For Charlie, more than anything, I wanted him to simply be more
aware of his choices. And though I may have failed in my judgment-free
facilitation of that awareness, it did have a positive impact.

Perhaps losing a parent to disease was an implicit motivator, but once
the New Year arrived, it was Charlie who was in resolution mode. And
though I wanted to come out on the other side of my project without the

need for rules and regulations, I decided to be his accountability buddy. If Charlie limited his red meat to once a week, I would recommit to my thirty minutes of movement. And we both would create some safeguards around our alcohol consumption, including another liver reset in February and a dry week every month. We also committed to the spirit of adventure, embracing the novelty of our neighborhood together, and relished in the fact that it somehow contained no Thai restaurants.

SO AM I FULLY HEALED? Have I found the magic recipe for healthy hedonism that allows me to feel good while indulging in all life's pleasures? Ah, how I wish.

"The real coming to terms with autoimmune disease is recognizing that you are sick, that the sickness will come and go, and that it is often not the kind of sick you can conquer," wrote fellow Hashimoto's sufferer Meghan O'Rourke in *The New Yorker*.

My year reminded me what my body was truly capable of. And my new normal is one that makes me feel happy and at ease in my own skin. But I still have bad days. When you're sensitive, it doesn't take much to knock you back a few steps. And I may never feel 100 percent without some sacrifices I'm unwilling to make.

Though my project is over, there never really was a finish line. The questioning doesn't end. As more products, studies, and solutions hit the market, my carefully crafted intuition becomes ever more valuable. Like a charcoal stick for the soul.

I'm stuck with the body I've got, faulty thyroid, gangly limbs, and all. To keep my judgment in line (toward myself and others), I try to remember that awareness is the first, and perhaps the most important, step toward healthy hedonism. Forgiveness is the second.

You have to stop fighting your body before it can stop fighting itself.

We all put one foot in front of the other and do the best we can. And for those of us lucky enough to take the scenic route around Health Mountain, I can attest to the awe and humility you experience when you take a step back, look over the edge, and marvel at how far you've come.

Change isn't easy. There is no hack. You cannot do it with a like or retweet, or through a sachet of detox tea and a twenty-day diet.

As Acu Heidi put it: healing isn't for pussies.

Every day forces me to find a new balance. To choose what goes on either side of the scale. A pat of butter on one, some chia seeds on the other. A margarita with a side of dancing. A pre-bedtime blue light–filled TV marathon, my hand intertwined with the hand of the man I love.

I know which of my choices might cause downstream harm. And I know when to ignore them in favor of living.

Because there's grace in the freedom of imperfection.

And after all, tomorrow there will always be more kale.

APPENDICES

The Golden Rules of Designing Your Own Health Odyssey

Instead of resolutions this year, I encourage you to make a list of short-term health challenges. You can take on these experiments monthly or weekly, making the total timeline as short or as long as you'd like. The goal is to get to know yourself better: what feeds your mind, body, and spirit; what changes make a profound difference and which might not be worth your time. At the end of your project, my hope is that you'll have figured out a better way forward. Because we can't commit to our good health habits until we discover what habits are actually good for us in the first place.

Here are five golden rules to keep in mind:

1. Build your wellness brain trust. This doesn't necessarily have to be made up of practitioners who you pay by the hour, but having a trusted physician is essential for any health undertaking. Your team could include a few expert voices from afar, and even some nonexpert friendly faces who can serve as accountability buddies and sounding boards. Listen to what they say with a grain of salt and filter their advice through your own experience.

2. Make your biggest intention to pay attention. The proof is in the pudding, and oftentimes your poop. Keep track of your body, whether through a journal, chart, app, or calendar. And don't just record numbers and symptoms: also check in with your spirit.

3. *Find power in the present.* Research has shown that immediate rewards are often more compelling than long-term gains. Recognize the positive outcomes that are tangible in the moment. They will help you commit to habits in the future.

4. *Give yourself permission to fail.* Change is hard work, and sometimes it takes periods of extremity to get to a place of balance. But as you try new things, remember that just because something worked for someone else doesn't mean it's going to work for you. Ask exactly what is making you uncomfortable and give yourself the leeway to pull the plug.

5. *Remember that perfection is a myth.* Awareness is the first and most important step toward healthy hedonism. Forgiveness is the second. We're all just doing the best we can.

The Healthy Hedonist Ten Commandments

1. Control your blood sugar.

2. Detox your product pantry.

3. Make your plate at least 50 percent veggies.

4. Cook the majority of your meals.

5. Drink cleaner water and more of it.

6. Move for thirty minutes every day.

7. Allow yourself time to rest.

8. One edible probiotic a day keeps the doctor away.

9. Use your mind as medicine.

10. Create a healthy home; find flexibility out in the world.

My Ten Best Wellness Buys

1. Green Skin-Care Products (see "My Everyday Bathroom Cabinet" below for the full list)

2. New Wave Enviro 10-Stage Water Filter

3. Kishu Binchotan Charcoal Sticks

4. Pelican 3-Stage Shower Filter

5. ClassPass Membership (1 Month)

6. CBT for Insomnia Conquering Insomnia Program

7. uBiome Gut Kit

8. Thrive Market Membership (1 Year)

9. mStand Laptop Stand

10. Vedic Meditation Training

My Everyday Bathroom Cabinet

• Evan Healy Blue Chamomile Moisturizer ($40)

• Evan Healy Blue Lavender Cleansing Milk ($30)

• Dr. Bronner's Magic All-One Organic Virgin Coconut Oil ($20)

• Dr. Bronner's Peppermint Pure-Castile Liquid Soap ($10)

• 100 Percent Pure Burdock and Neem Healthy Scalp Shampoo and Conditioner ($20, $25)

• Dr. Hauschka Foundation ($38)

• W3LL People Universalist Multi-Stick Blush ($35)

- Jane Iredale Eye Pencil ($15)
- Abbey St Clare Concealer ($18)
- Babo Botanicals Clear Zinc Sunscreen Lotion ($20)
- Blissoma Scentless Stick Natural Deodorant ($15)

My bathroom cabinet is constantly changing as I find new amazing green products. For more up-to-date suggestions and purchasing information, visit FeedMePhoebe.com/Shop.

The Best Green Beauty Boutiques and Retailers

Ayla*
  http://aylabeauty.com

Beau Tea Bar*
  http://www.beauteabar.com

BeautyKind
  https://beautykind.us

Bella Floria Organics
  http://www.bellafloria.com

Blades Natural Beauty
  http://bladesnaturalbeauty.bigcartel.com

CAP Beauty*
  http://www.capbeauty.com

The Choosy Chick
  http://thechoosychick.com

Credo*
  http://credobeauty.com

The Detox Market*
  http://www.thedetoxmarket.com

EcoDiva

https://www.ecodivabeauty.com

Follain*

http://shopfollain.com

LeVert Beauty

https://levertbeauty.com

Pharmaca*

http://www.pharmaca.com

Shen Beauty*

http://www.shen-beauty.com

Spirit Beauty Lounge

http://www.spiritbeautylounge.com

The Truth Beauty Company

http://www.thetruthbeautycompany.com

*Select brick-and-mortar locations available.

My Favorite Health Apps

• Think Dirty

• Environmental Working Group's Healthy Living (Skin Deep)

• Moro

• My Pilates Guru

• YogaGlo

• f.lux

• Kindara

• Tummy Trends

• Insight Timer

• Headspace

Five Tips for Your Farmer's Market Batch-Cooking Challenge

This challenge involves setting aside one weekend to cook meals for the week ahead. It can be done anywhere, including the regular grocery store. The idea is to give yourself a set budget (mine was forty dollars) and to spend that money solely on fresh produce, meat, and seafood. If you're not shopping from small farms, try to buy organic or use the Environmental Working Group's Clean Fifteen list to avoid pesticide-heavy produce. To keep costs down, focus on buying less meat (one pound per week at most), filling in the gaps with whole grains and other pantry ingredients (especially your spice rack!), and avoiding unnecessary items that you won't use start to finish.

Design your menu around four or five recipes and keep in mind that each dish should:

1. Include at least one fresh veggie or fruit (duh).

2. Be simple enough to be prepared in a weekend afternoon.

3. Last for several days (stews, soups, grains, stir-fries, and roasted veggies keep better than raw).

4. Use a different cooking technique for each dish—a mix of roasting, sautéing, and raw—instead of making four dishes that require the stovetop or oven.

5. Adhere to the same cuisine so you can mix and match throughout the week. You'll also save money if the same herbs can be used in several dishes.

Sample Menus

Check out each recipe's Market Swap notes for more ways to vary the seasonal produce.

Fall/Winter

Turmeric-Braised Chicken Legs with Golden Beets and Leeks *(page 190)*

Chili-Roasted Root Vegetables with Chickpeas, Tahini, and Brazil Nut Pangritata *(page 274)*

Marinated Kale with Tamari-Roasted Beets and Sesame Seeds (omit beets) *(page 277)*

Desperation Minestrone Soup *(page 131)*

Spring/Summer

Almond-Sesame Soba Zoodles with Quick Pickled Veggies *(page 332)*

Shrimp and Asparagus Pesto Pasta Salad with Chives *(page 308)*

Vegan Quinoa "Fried Rice" with Rainbow Chard *(page 103)*

Grilled Romaine Hearts with Roasted Shallots, Artichoke Hearts, and Kefir Green Goddess Dressing *(page 305)*

Recipe Index

BREAKFAST

Dad's Overnight Oatmeal with Almond Butter and Dried Cherries *(page 243)*

Golden Milk Chia Pudding with Cinnamon Yogurt *(page 188)*

Green Egg (No Ham) Frittata Bites *(page 218)*

Violet's Big Blueberry-Almond Smoothie *(page 46)*

SOUPS AND SALADS

Desperation Minestrone Soup *(page 131)*

Grilled Romaine Hearts with Roasted Shallots, Artichoke Hearts, and
  Kefir Green Goddess Dressing *(page 305)*

Marinated Kale with Tamari-Roasted Beets and Sesame Seeds *(page 277)*

"Pho Real" Slow Cooker Ginger-Chicken Bone Broth *(page 165)*

Vietnamese Chicken Soup for the Soul *(page 330)*

MAINS

Almond-Sesame Soba Zoodles with Quick Pickled Veggies *(page 332)*

Chili-Roasted Root Vegetables with Chickpeas, Tahini, and Brazil Nut
  Pangritata *(page 274)*

Shrimp and Asparagus Pesto Pasta Salad with Chives *(page 308)*

Skillet Red-Wine Braised Cabbage and Lentils *(page 133)*

Turmeric-Braised Chicken Legs with Golden Beets and Leeks *(page 190)*

Vegan Quinoa "Fried Rice" with Rainbow Chard *(page 103)*

SIDES AND SNACKS

Baked Sweet Potato Fries with Coconut Oil–Sriracha Aioli *(page 105)*

Raw Gingerbread Cookie Beauty Balls *(page 78)*

Sweet and Spicy Pepita-Cashew Snack Mix *(page 76)*

Thai Peanut Humus with Farmer's Market Crudités *(page 220)*

DRINKS

Ginger-Lime Ice Cubes *(page 160)*

Green Tea Arnold Palmers *(page 48)*

Sleepy Tummy Tea *(page 245)*

ACKNOWLEDGMENTS

The following people made many appearances in my gratitude journal, and this book is truly a product of their many talents, tireless work, gracious hand-holding, and constant cheerleading.

An all-encompassing thank you to Sally Ekus, for being an excellent eavesdropper and having the chutzpah to tap me on the shoulder at a coffee shop in the East Village and ask me what I did in the food world. I am endlessly grateful to the benevolent force that made this chance encounter happen, and to you for riding the wave of my many wacky ideas until they led here. I feel so fortunate to call you my agent and, better yet, my friend.

To Pam Krauss for taking a gamble on this newbie author and welcoming my project as an early member of your family of books. I'm so lucky to have had an editor who gave me plenty of freedom to roam and, five hundred pages later, knew how to tactfully reel me in. This book is infinitely better as a result of your wisdom. And for preventing me from starting every third sentence with "And."

To Nina Caldas, Casey Maloney, Roshe Anderson, and the rest of the Avery/Penguin Random House team for embracing this book and shepherding it into the world.

To Julia Taylor-Brown, whose illustrations brought the pages to life, made me LOL on multiple occasions, and served as their own special dose of "life pills" for this isolated writer.

To all the institutions and individuals who gave me a quiet, safe space to concentrate, retreat from the world, take wine-filled baths, and not shower for days on end: Rivendell Writers' Colony, Writing Between the Vines, Maderas Village, and Denny and Barbara Kernochan, who had the most delicious California cuisine of any retreat.

To my wellness brain trust: Kristen Arnett, Cindy DiPrima, Kerri-lynn Pamer, Jessa Blades, Dr. Amy Wechsler, Leanne Brown, Juliet Maris, Alisa Vitti, Katinka Locascio, Dr. Robynne Chutkan, Erica and Justin Sonnenburg, Dr. Robin Berzin, Nichola Weir, Amie Valpone, and Ben Turshen, who shared their wisdom with me, and help countless other people on their wellness journeys every day. And a special thank-you to Heidi Lovie, the wisest woman I know, whose advice flows through every page of this book. You saved me from myself, and for that, gratitude courses through every inch of my heart meridian.

To my behind-the-scenes edit team: Allie White for your whip-smart questions and encyclopedic knowledge of green beauty; Kate Rosenblatt and Michaela Motta for your early information mining; Whitney Toombs, Steph Malloch, Payal Khurana, Liz Presson, Allison Kade, and Caitlyn Fox for your feedback on early drafts.

To my chosen family: the dozens of friends who read sections, let me pick their brains on various wellness practices, and talked me off the ledge before I started meditating. In particular, Sarah Stein-Sapir for attempting to impart your fitness prowess on me, and Sarah Brown for holding my hand at the doctor's office, and introducing me to a fahncy fella to take over those duties.

To Debbie Phillips and Cheryl Houser for your mentorship, Amber Rae and the Alive Tribe for making me get on a table and (almost) believe that I was a writer. Your collective confidence in the message of this book is a huge reason it got written.

To KC Baker and Jill Tyler for helping me share my voice, Leslie Zaikis for your brilliant launch advice, and Stacie Kenton and Amy English for keeping all my other food ventures afloat while I was off the grid writing.

To the readers of *Feed Me Phoebe* (especially Frankie) for all your virtual encouragement, compassionate typo feedback, and for simply showing up. Anytime you comment or post about a recipe you've made, it's like drinking an unparalleled smoothie of endorphins, dopamine, and serotonin. Thank you for sharing your own health struggles and making me feel that I wasn't alone in mine. And big-time gratitude to my Healthy Hedonist Guinea Pig Group for your eagerness to be part of the challenges, and for your forgiveness when I realized I didn't have the bandwidth to support you and write a book at the same time.

To my stepson, Baron the Beagle. If there was a humane and shed-free way to make a blanket from your velvety ears, I would. But I'll settle for getting to pet them every day. Thank you for your unconditional doggy love, lessons in parenting, and tireless composting of my kale and broccoli stems. The house feels clean but empty without you.

To my dad, for modeling creativity as lifeblood, and for showing me that being a successful writer takes hard work, commitment to the editing process, and a lot of chocolate. You've always pushed me to pursue my dreams, be more generous, and eat the occasional dessert. Art isn't easy, but your support has made me careful not to lose the way.

To my mom, for reading Every. Single. Draft, with feedback that always struck the perfect balance of kind and constructive. You're the most brilliant person I know, and I feel so lucky that 1 percent of those genes trickled down to me. Thank you for putting your love on the plate (and veal scallopini in the blender) from day one, for showing me how to meditate over a pan of caramelizing onions, and for being the first investor in Phoebe's Restaurant, and its biggest supporter ever since.

And, finally, to Charlie for being by my side for every step of this process, even when I disappeared for weeks on end into the WiFi-less wilderness, and for your endless patience, calming mid-meltdown demeanor, and willingness to let me share so many snapshots of our life together. You're truly the best thing that ever happened to my health and hedonism, and I thank my lucky stars every day for the Fourth of July fireworks that have been going off in my chest ever since I (re)met you.

BIBLIOGRAPHY

PREFACE: FROM FEEDING ON FADS TO FINDING "BALANCE"

American Psychological Association. "Making Lifestyle Changes That Last." http://www.apa.org/helpcenter/lifestyle-changes.aspx

Dingfelder, Sadie. "Solutions to Resolution Dilution." *American Psychological Association*, January 2004; 35.1 (January 2004): 34. http://www.apa.org/monitor/jan04/solutions.aspx

Rubin, Gretchen. *The Happiness Project: Or Why I Spent a Year Trying to Sing in the Morning, Clean My Closets, Fight Right, Read Aristotle, and Generally Have More Fun*. New York: Harper, 2009.

DRUNK IN LOVE . . . WITH MY LIVER: THE VICE DETOX

Alpert, Brooke, and Patricia Farris. *The Sugar Detox: Lose Weight, Feel Great, and Look Years Younger*. Boston: Da Capo Lifelong, 2013.

The American Heart Association. "Sugar 101." http://www.heart.org/HEARTORG/HealthyLiving/HealthyEating/Nutrition/Sugar-101_UCM_306024_Article.jsp#.WF7FwDKZPVo

Boekema, P.J., M. Samsom, and G. P. Van Be. "Coffee and Gastrointestinal Function: Facts and Fiction: A Review." *Scandinavian Journal of Gastroenterology* 34.230 (1999): 35–39. http://www.ncbi.nlm.nih.gov/pubmed/10499460

Hyman, Mark. *The Blood Sugar Solution: The Ultrahealthy Program for Losing Weight, Preventing Disease, and Feeling Great Now!* New York: Little, Brown, 2012.

Jakubowicz, Daniela, Julio Wainstein, Bo Ahren, Zohar Landau, Yosefa Bar-Dayan, and Oren Froy. "Fasting Until Noon Triggers Increased Postprandial Hyperglycemia and Impaired Insulin Response After Lunch and Dinner in Individuals with Type 2 Diabetes: A Randomized Clinical Trial." *Diabetes Care* 38.10 (October 2015): 1820–826. http://care.diabetesjournals.org /content/38/10/1820

Lenoir, Magalie, Fuschia Serre, Lauriane Cantin, and Serge H. Ahmed. "Intense Sweetness Surpasses Cocaine Reward." *PLoS ONE* 2.8 (2007). https://www .ncbi.nlm.nih.gov/pubmed/17668074

Lucero, Jennifer, Bernard L. Harlow, Robert L. Barbieri, Patrick Sluss, and Daniel W. Cramer. "Early Follicular Phase Hormone Levels in Relation to Patterns of Alcohol, Tobacco, and Coffee Use." *Fertility and Sterility* 76.4 (2001): 723–29. https://www.ncbi.nlm.nih.gov/pubmed/11591405

Patwardhan, R.V., P. Desmond, R. Johnson, and S. Schenker. "Impaired Elimination of Caffeine by Oral Contraceptive Steroids." *The Journal of Laboratory and Clinical Medicine* 95.4 (April 1980): 603–8. https://www.ncbi.nlm.nih.gov /pubmed/7359014

Stephanie Soechtig, director, *Fed Up*. The Weinstein Company, 2014.

Yang, Amy, Abraham A. Palmer, and Harriet De Wit. "Genetics of Caffeine Consumption and Responses to Caffeine." *Psychopharmacology* 211.3 (August 2010): 245–57. https://www.ncbi.nlm.nih.gov/pmc/articles/PMC4242593/

GREEN BEAUTY: FEEDING MY SKIN FROM THE OUTSIDE IN

Altemus, Margaret, Babar Rao, Firdaus S. Dhabhar, Wanhong Ding, and Richard D. Granstein. "Stress-Induced Changes in Skin Barrier Function in Healthy Women." *Journal of Investigative Dermatology* 117.2 (August 2001): 309–17. https://www.ncbi.nlm.nih.gov/pubmed/11511309

Barr, L., G. Metaxas, C. A. J. Harbach, L. A. Savoy, and P. D. Darbre. "Measurement of Paraben Concentrations in Human Breast Tissue at Serial Locations across the Breast from Axilla to Sternum." *Journal of Applied Toxicology* 32.3 (March 2012): 219–32. https://www.ncbi.nlm.nih.gov/pubmed/22237600

Cha, Hwa Jun, Seunghee Bae, Karam Kim, Seung Bin Kwon, In-Sook An, Kyu Joong Ahn, Junghwa Ryu, Hey-Sun Kim, Sang-Kyu Ye, Byung-Hak Kim, and Sungkwan An. "Overdosage of Methylparaben Induces Cellular

Senescence In Vitro and In Vivo." *Journal of Investigative Dermatology* 135.2 (February 2015): 609–12. https://www.ncbi.nlm.nih.gov/pubmed/25229254

Chakraborty, Tandra, Eilliut Alicea, and Sanjoy Chakraborty. "Relationships between Urinary Biomarkers of Phytoestrogens, Phthalates, Phenols, and Pubertal Stages in Girls." *Adolescent Health, Medicine and Therapeutics* 3 (January 2012): 17. https://www.ncbi.nlm.nih.gov/pubmed/20308033

DiGangi, Joseph, Ted Schettler, Madeleine Cobbing, and Mark Rossi. *Aggregate Exposures to Phthalates in Humans.* Washington, DC: Health Care Without Harm, 2002. http://www.fda.gov/ohrms/dockets/dailys/02/Dec02/120502 /02d-0325-c000018-02-vol1.pdf

Duhigg, Charles. *The Power of Habit: Why We Do What We Do in Life and Business.* New York: Random House, 2012.

Environmental Working Group. "Skin Deep® Cosmetics Database." http://www .ewg.org/skindeep/

Grigore, Adina. *Skin Cleanse: The Simple, All-Natural Program for Clear, Calm, Happy Skin.* New York: HarperWave, 2015.

Marati, Jessica. "What You Need to Know About Aveda's Natural Ingredients." *EcoSalon.* March 30, 2012. http://ecosalon.com/behind-the-label-aveda -natural-beauty-products/

Safe Cosmetics website. "Campaign for Safe Cosmetics." http://www.safecosmet ics.org

Vitello, Paul. "Horst Rechelbacher, 'Father of Safe Cosmetics,' Dies at 72." *The New York Times.* February 22, 2014. http://www.nytimes.com/2014/02/23 /business/horst-rechelbacher-father-of-safe-cosmetics-dies-at-72.html?_r=0

Wechsler, Amy. *The Mind-Beauty Connection: 9 Days to Reverse Stress Aging and Reveal More Youthful, Beautiful Skin.* New York: Free Press, 2008.

Wolfer, Alexis. *The Recipe for Radiance: Discover Beauty's Best-Kept Secrets in Your Kitchen.* Philadelphia: Running Press, 2014.

GUT GUILT: EATING WITHOUT ABANDON

American Autoimmune Related Diseases Association website. https://www .aarda.org

Barboza, David. "In China, Farming Fish in Toxic Waters." *The New York Times.* December 15, 2007. http://www.nytimes.com/2007/12/15/world/asia /15fish.html?hp')

Bi, William. "Asian Seafood Raised on Pig Feces Approved for U.S. Consumers." *Bloomberg Markets.* October 11, 2012. http://www.bloomberg.com/news /articles/2012-10-11/asian-seafood-raised-on-pig-feces-approved -for-u-s-consumers

Bittman, Mark. *VB6: Eat Vegan Before 6:00 to Lose Weight and Restore Your Health . . . for Good.* New York: Clarkson Potter, 2013.

Blum, Susan S., and Michele Bender. *The Immune System Recovery Plan: A Doctor's 4-Step Program to Treat Autoimmune Disease.* New York: Scribner, 2013.

Buettner, Dan. *The Blue Zones Solution: Eating and Living like the World's Healthiest People.* Washington, DC: National Geographic, 2015.

Carr, Kris. *Crazy Sexy Cancer Tips.* Guilford, CT: Skirt!, 2007.

Dean, Tommy. "Why 160 Countries Say 'No' to US Meat." *Veg News.* March 14, 2013. http://vegnews.com/articles/page.do?pageId=5537&catId=1

Frazier, Karen. *The Hashimoto's 4-Week Plan: A Holistic Guide to Treating Hypothyroidism.* Berkeley: Sonoma Press, 2016.

Fromartz, Samuel. "The Gluten Enigma." *Eating Well.* March/April 2015. http:// www.eatingwell.com/nutrition_health/nutrition_news_information/unravel ing_the_gluten_free_trend?socsrc=ewtw0224152

Hamblin, James. "This Is Your Brain on Gluten." *The Atlantic.* December 20, 2013. http://www.theatlantic.com/health/archive/2013/12/this-is-your -brain-on-gluten/282550/

IARC Monographs Evaluate Consumption of Red Meat and Processed Meat. World Health Organization, 2015. http://www.iarc.fr/en/media-centre/pr/2015/pdfs /pr240_E.pdf

Kimble, Megan. *Unprocessed: My City-Dwelling Year of Reclaiming Real Food.* New York: William Morrow, 2015.

Lipman, Frank, and Danielle Claro. *The New Health Rules: Simple Changes to Achieve Whole-Body Wellness.* New York: Artisan, 2014.

Perlmutter, David, and Kristin Loberg. *Grain Brain: The Surprising Truth About Wheat, Carbs, and Sugar—Your Brain's Silent Killers.* New York: Little, Brown and Company, 2013.

Robbins, John. *The Food Revolution: How Your Diet Can Help Save Your Life and Our World.* Berkeley: Conari Press, 2001.

Specter, Michael. "Against the Grain." *The New Yorker.* November 3, 2014. http:// www.newyorker.com/magazine/2014/11/03/grain

Villarica, Hans. "The Chocolate-and-Radish Experiment That Birthed the Modern Conception of Willpower." *The Atlantic.* April 9, 2012. http://www .theatlantic.com/health/archive/2012/04/the-chocolate-and-radish -experiment-that-birthed-the-modern-conception-of-willpower/255544/

SKILLET SKILLS: BECOMING MY OWN PERSONAL CHEF

Bowen, Sarah, Sinikka Elliott, and Joslyn Brenton. "The Joy of Cooking?" *Contexts.* August 22, 2014: 20–25. http://contexts.org/articles/the-joy-of-cooking/

Brown, Leanne. *Good and Cheap: Eat Well on $4/Day.* New York: Workman, 2015.

Dog, Tieraona Low. *Fortify Your Life: Your Guide to Vitamins, Minerals, and More.* Washington, DC: National Geographic, 2016.

Environmental Working Group. "EWG's 2016 Shopper's Guide to Pesticides in Produce™." https://www.ewg.org/foodnews/summary.php

Havermans, Remco C., and Anita Jansen. "Increasing Children's Liking of Vegetables through Flavour–Flavour Learning." *Appetite* 48.2 (March 2007): 259–62. https://www.ncbi.nlm.nih.gov/pubmed/17113192

Holt-Lunstad, Julianne, Timothy Smith, and J. Layton. "Social Relationships and Mortality Risk: A Meta-Analytic Review." *PloS Med* 7.7 (July 2010). http:// journals.plos.org/plosmedicine/article?id=10.1371/journal.pmed.1000316#top

Hyman, Mark. *Eat Fat, Get Thin: Why the Fat We Eat Is the Key to Sustained Weight Loss and Vibrant Health.* New York: Little, Brown and Company, 2016.

Lakkakula, Anantha, James Geaghan, Michael Zanovec, Sarah Pierce, and Georgianna Tuuri. "Repeated Taste Exposure Increases Liking for Vegetables by Low-Income Elementary School Children." *Appetite* 55.2 (October 2010): 226–31. https://www.ncbi.nlm.nih.gov/pubmed/20541572

Lu, J., C. Huet, and L. Dube. "Emotional Reinforcement as a Protective Factor for Healthy Eating in Home Settings." *American Journal of Clinical Nutrition* 94.1 (July 2011): 254–61. https://www.ncbi.nlm.nih.gov/pubmed/21613564

Myers, Amy. *The Autoimmune Solution: Prevent and Reverse the Full Spectrum of Inflammatory Symptoms and Diseases.* San Francisco: HarperOne, 2015.

Pollan, Michael. *Food Rules: An Eater's Manual.* New York: Penguin, 2009.

United States Department of Agriculture Economic Research Service. "Percent of consumer expenditures spent on food, alcoholic beverages, and tobacco that were consumed at home, by selected countries, 2014." https://www.ers.usda .gov/data-products/food-expenditures.aspx

Wolfson, Julia A., and Sara N. Bleich. "Is Cooking at Home Associated with Better Diet Quality or Weight-loss Intention?" *Public Health Nutrition* 18.8 (November 2014): 1397–406. https://www.cambridge.org/core/journals /public-health-nutrition/article/div-classtitleis-cooking-at-home-associated -with-better-diet-quality-or-weight-loss-intentiondiv/ B2C8C168FFA377DD2880A217DB6AF26F

Worldwatch Institute. "Is Meat Sustainable?" *World Watch Magazine* 17.4 (July 2004). http://www.worldwatch.org/node/549

WATER WORKS: FILLING MY WELL

The Associated Press. "Cleveland Takes Offense at Fiji Water Ad." *The Washington Post.* July 20, 2006. http://www.washingtonpost.com/wp-dyn/content/article /2006/07/20/AR2006072000322.html

Batmanghelidj, F. *Water: For Health, for Healing, for Life: You're Not Sick, You're Thirsty!* New York: Warner, 2003.

Batmanghelidj, F. *Your Body's Many Cries for Water.* Virginia: Global Health Solutions, 1997.

Blau, Joseph Norman, Christian Alexander Kell, and Julia Maria Sperling. "Water-Deprivation Headache: A New Headache with Two Variants." *Headache: The Journal of Head and Face Pain* 44.1 (January 2004): 79–83. https://www.ncbi.nlm.nih.gov/pubmed/14979888

Carroll, Aaron E. "Simple Rules for Healthy Eating." *The New York Times.* April 20, 2015. http://www.nytimes.com/2015/04/21/upshot/simple-rules-for -healthy-eating.html?smid=nytcore-iphone-share&smprod=nytcore-iphone& _r=0&abt=0002&abg=0

Collins, Danica. "Dangers of Chlorine in Your Shower." *Underground Health Reporter.* July 13, 2011. http://undergroundhealthreporter.com /dangers-of-chlorine-in-your-shower/

Donn, Jeff, Martha Mendoza, and Justin Pritchard. "Pharmaceuticals Found in Drinking Water, Affecting Wildlife and Maybe Humans." The Associated Press. 2008. http://hosted.ap.org/specials/interactives/pharmawater_site/day1 _01.html

Duhigg, Charles. "That Tap Water Is Legal but May Be Unhealthy." *The New York Times.* December 16, 2009. http://www.nytimes.com/2009/12/17/us /17water.html

Fallik, Dawn. "This New Study Found More Drugs in Our Drinking Water Than Anybody Knew." *The New Republic*. December 11, 2013. https://newrepublic.com/article/115883/drugs-drinking-water-new-epa-study-finds-more-we-knew

Kalman, Douglas S., Samantha Feldman, Diane R. Krieger, and Richard J. Bloomer. "Comparison of Coconut Water and a Carbohydrate-Electrolyte Sport Drink on Measures of Hydration and Physical Performance in Exercise-Trained Men." *Journal of the International Society of Sports Nutrition* 9.1 (January 2012). http://jissn.biomedcentral.com/articles/10.1186/1550-2783-9-1

Kenney, Erica L., Michael W. Long, Angie L. Cradock, and Steven L. Gortmaker. "Prevalence of Inadequate Hydration Among US Children and Disparities by Gender and Race/Ethnicity: National Health and Nutrition Examination Survey, 2009–2012." *American Journal of Public Health* 105.8 (January 2015). http://ajph.aphapublications.org/doi/abs/10.2105/AJPH.2015.302572

Kurlansky, Mark. *Salt: A World History*. New York: Walker, 2002.

Moss, Michael. "Coconut Water Changes Its Claims." *The New York Times*. July 26, 2014. http://www.nytimes.com/2014/07/30/dining/coconut-water-changes-its-claims.html?_r=0

Watson, Phillip, Andrew Whale, Stephen A. Mears, Louise A. Reyner, and Ronald J. Maughan. "Mild Hypohydration Increases the Frequency of Driver Errors during a Prolonged, Monotonous Driving Task." *Physiology & Behavior* 147 (August 2015): 313–18. http://www.sciencedirect.com/science/article/pii/S0031938415002358

BACK IT UP: CHIRO-PRACTICAL PHYSICAL THERAPY

Booth, Frank W., Christian K. Roberts, and Matthew J. Laye. "Lack of Exercise Is a Major Cause of Chronic Diseases." *Comprehensive Physiology* 2.2 (April 2012): 1143–1211. https://www.ncbi.nlm.nih.gov/pmc/articles/PMC4241367/

MacEwen, Brittany T., Dany J. Macdonald, and Jamie F. Burr. "A Systematic Review of Standing and Treadmill Desks in the Workplace." *Preventive Medicine* 70 (January 2015): 50–58. https://www.ncbi.nlm.nih.gov/pubmed/25448843

Oppezzo, Marily, and Daniel L. Schwartz. "Give Your Ideas Some Legs: The Positive Effect of Walking on Creative Thinking." *Journal of Experimental Psychology: Learning, Memory, and Cognition* 40.4 (July 2014): 1142–152. https://www.ncbi.nlm.nih.gov/pubmed/24749966

Relieving Pain in America: A Blueprint for Transforming Prevention, Care, Education, and Research. Washington, DC: Institute of Medicine, 2011. http://www .nationalacademies.org/hmd/Reports/2011/Relieving-Pain-in-America-A -Blueprint-for-Transforming-Prevention-Care-Education-Research/Report -Brief.aspx

Sadeghi, Habib. "Emotional Erosion and Uncontained Anger." *Goop.* March 12, 2015. http://goop.com/emotional-erosion-and-uncontained-anger/

Sarno, John E. *Healing Back Pain: The Mind-Body Connection.* New York: Warner, 1991.

Veerman, J. Lennert, Genevieve N. Healy, Linda J. Cobiac, Theo Vos, Elisabeth A. H. Winkler, Neville Owen, and David W. Dunstan. "Television Viewing Time and Reduced Life Expectancy: A Life Table Analysis." *British Journal of Sports Medicine* 46.3 (October 2012): 927–30. https://www.ncbi.nlm.nih.gov /pubmed/23007179

Wilson, Sarah. "Could female self-hatred be the real cause of autoimmune disease?" SarahWilson.com. November 18, 2014. http://www.sarahwilson .com/2014/11/could-female-self-hatred-be-the-real-cause-of-autoimmune -disease/

Wittman, Jen. *Healing Hashimoto's Naturally: How I Used Radical TLC to Love My Thyroid and My Body Back to Health . . . and You Can Too!* United States: Healthy Plate, LLC, 2014.

MAKING MOVES: FITTING FITNESS INTO EVERYDAY LIFE

Arem, Hannah, Steven C. Moore, Alpa Patel, Patricia Hartge, Amy Berrington De Gonzalez, Kala Visvanathan, Peter T. Campbell, Michal Freedman, Elisabete Weiderpass, Hans Olov Adami, Martha S. Linet, I.-Min Lee, and Charles E. Matthews. "Leisure Time Physical Activity and Mortality: A Detailed Pooled Analysis of the Dose-Response Relationship." *JAMA Internal Medicine* 175.6 (June 2015): 959. https://www.ncbi.nlm.nih.gov/pubmed /25844730

Bowman, Katy. *Move Your DNA: Restore Your Health through Natural Movement.* Carlsborg, WA: Propriometrics Press, 2014.

Bravata, Dena M., Crystal Smith-Spangler, Vandana Sundaram, Allison L. Gienger, Nancy Lin, Robyn Lewis, Christopher D. Stave, Ingram Olkin, and John R. Sirard. "Using Pedometers to Increase Physical Activity and Improve Health." *JAMA* 298.19 (November 2007): 2296. https://www.ncbi.nlm.nih .gov/pubmed/18029834

Brito, L. B. B. De, D. R. Ricardo, D. S. M. S. De Araújo, P. S. Ramos, J. Myers, and C. G. S. De Araujo. "Ability to Sit and Rise from the Floor as a Predictor of All-Cause Mortality." *European Journal of Preventive Cardiology* 21.7 (July 2012). https://www.ncbi.nlm.nih.gov/pubmed/23242910

Ferriss, Timothy. *The 4-Hour Body: An Uncommon Guide to Rapid Fat Loss, Incredible Sex, and Becoming Superhuman.* New York: Harmony, 2010.

Harvard School of Public Healthy. "Obesity Prevention Source." https://www.hsph.harvard.edu/obesity-prevention-source/moderate-and-vigorous-physical-activity/

Jacobs, A. J. *Drop Dead Healthy: One Man's Humble Quest for Bodily Perfection.* New York: Simon & Schuster, 2012.

Lincoln, Sadie. *Love Your Lower Body: The 8-Week Plan to Sculpt a Slender, Strong, and Beautiful Physique.* Emmaus, PA: Rodale, 2014.

McDougall, Christopher. *Born to Run: A Hidden Tribe, Superathletes, and the Greatest Race the World Has Never Seen.* New York: Knopf, 2009.

McDougall, Christopher. *Natural Born Heroes: How a Daring Band of Misfits Mastered the Lost Secrets of Strength and Endurance.* New York: Knopf, 2015.

McGonigal, Kelly. *The Willpower Instinct: How Self-Control Works, Why It Matters, and What You Can Do to Get More of It.* New York: Avery, 2011.

Rosenkilde, M., P. Auerbach, M. H. Reichkendler, T. Ploug, B. M. Stallknecht, and A. Sjödin. "Body Fat Loss and Compensatory Mechanisms in Response to Different Doses of Aerobic Exercise—A Randomized Controlled Trial in Overweight Sedentary Males." *AJP: Regulatory, Integrative and Comparative Physiology* 303.6 (September 2012). https://www.ncbi.nlm.nih.gov/pubmed/22855277

Rubin, Gretchen. *Better than Before: Mastering the Habits of Our Everyday Lives.* New York: Crown, 2015.

Segar, Michelle. *No Sweat: How the Simple Science of Motivation Can Bring You a Lifetime of Fitness.* New York: AMACOM, 2015.

PILLOW TALK: HITTING THE SNOOZE BUTTON

CBT for Insomnia. http://www.cbtforinsomnia.com

Frakt, Austin. "The Evidence Points to a Better Way to Fight Insomnia." *The New York Times.* June 8, 2015. http://www.nytimes.com/2015/06/09/upshot/the-evidence-points-to-a-better-way-to-fight-insomnia.html

Gage, S. Billioti De, Y. Moride, T. Ducruet, T. Kurth, H. Verdoux, M. Tournier, A. Pariente, and B. Begaud. "Benzodiazepine Use and Risk of Alzheimer's Disease: Case-Control Study." *British Medical Journal* 349 (September 2014). http://www.bmj.com/content/349/bmj.g5205

Klösch, Gerhard, John Dittami, and Josef Zeitlhofer. *Sleeping Better Together: How Both of You Can Get a Better Night's Rest*. Alameda, CA: Hunter House, 2011.

Han, Emily. *Wild Drinks & Cocktails: Handcrafted Squashes, Shrubs, Switchels, Tonics, and Infusions to Mix at Home*. Beverly, MA: Fair Winds Press, 2015.

Huffington, Arianna. *Thrive: The Third Metric to Redefining Success and Creating a Life of Well-being, Wisdom, and Wonder*. New York: Harmony, 2014.

Ju, Yo-El S., Jennifer S. McLeland, Cristina D. Toedebusch, Chengjie Xiong, Anne M. Fagan, Stephen P. Duntley, John C. Morris, and David M. Holtzman. "Sleep Quality and Preclinical Alzheimer Disease." *JAMA Neurology* 70.5 (May 2013): 587. https://www.ncbi.nlm.nih.gov/pubmed/23479184

Palagini, Laura, Rosa Maria Bruno, Angelo Gemignani, Chiara Baglioni, Lorenzo Ghiadoni, and Dieter Riemann. "Sleep Loss and Hypertension: A Systematic Review." *Current Pharmaceutical Design* 19.13 (2013): 2409–419. https://www.ncbi.nlm.nih.gov/pubmed/23173590

Patel, Sanjay R., and Frank B. Hu. "Short Sleep Duration and Weight Gain: A Systematic Review." *Obesity* 16.3 (March 2008): 643–53. https://www.ncbi .nlm.nih.gov/pubmed/18239586

Risacher, Shannon L., Brenna C. McDonald, Eileen F. Tallman, John D. West, Martin R. Farlow, Fredrick W. Unverzagt, Sujuan Gao, Malaz Boustani, Paul K. Crane, Ronald C. Petersen, Clifford R. Jack, William J. Jagust, Paul S. Aisen, Michael W. Weiner, and Andrew J. Saykin. "Association Between Anticholinergic Medication Use and Cognition, Brain Metabolism, and Brain Atrophy in Cognitively Normal Older Adults." *JAMA Neurology* 73.6 (June 2016): 721. https://www.ncbi.nlm.nih.gov/pubmed/27088965

Rosenberg, Robert S. *Sleep Soundly Every Night, Feel Fantastic Every Day: A Doctor's Guide to Solving Your Sleep Problems*. New York: DemosHealth, 2014.

Sleep Deprivation Effect on the Immune System Mirrors Physical Stress. Darien, IL: American Academy of Sleep Medicine, 2012. http://www.aasmnet.org /articles.aspx?id=3196

Valpone, Annie. *Eating Clean: The 21-Day Plan to Detox, Fight Inflammation, and Reset Your Body*. New York: Houghton Mifflin Harcourt, 2016.

Van der Lely, Stephanie, Silvia Frey, Corrado Garbazza, Anna Wirz-Justice, Oskar G. Jenni, Roland Steiner, Stefan Wolf, Christian Cajochen, Vivien

Bromundt, and Christina Schmidt. "Blue Blocker Glasses as a Countermeasure for Alerting Effects of Evening Light-Emitting Diode Screen Exposure in Male Teenagers." *Journal of Adolescent Health* 56.1 (January 2015): 113–19. https://www.ncbi.nlm.nih.gov/pubmed/25287985

Vandewalle, Gilles, Olivier Collignon, Joseph T. Hull, Véronique Daneault, Geneviéve Albouy, Franco Lepore, Christophe Phillips, Julien Doyon, Charles A. Czeisler, Marie Dumont, Steven W. Lockley, and Julie Carrier. "Blue Light Stimulates Cognitive Brain Activity in Visually Blind Individuals." *Journal of Cognitive Neuroscience* 25.12 (October 2013): 2072–85. http://www.mitpressjournals.org/doi/abs/10.1162/jocn_a_00450# .WG5uIzKZPVo

RAG TIME: MOON SISTERHOOD AND THE STATE OF HORMONE HEALTH

Band, Emily. "How the Spoon Theory Helps Those Suffering Chronic Pain and Fatigue." *The Guardian*. September 24, 2012. https://www.theguardian.com /commentisfree/2012/sep/24/spoon-theory-chronic-pain-fatigue

Cooper, Trevor G., Elizabeth Noonan, Sigrid von Eckardstein, Jacques Auger, H.W. Gordon Baker, Hermann M. Behre, Trine B. Haugen, Thinus Kruger, Christina Wang, Michael T. Mvizvo, and Kirsten M. Vogelsong. "World Health Organization Reference Values for Human Semen Characteristics." *Human Reproduction Update* 16.3 (November 2009): 231–45. http://www.who .int/reproductivehealth/topics/infertility/cooper_et_al_hru.pdf

Finer, Lawrence B., and Mia R. Zolna. "Declines in Unintended Pregnancy in the United States, 2008–2011." *The New England Journal of Medicine* 374 (March 2016): 843–52. http://www.nejm.org/doi/full/10.1056/NEJMsa1506575

Friedman, Ann. "No Pill? No Prob. Meet the Pullout Generation." *New York Magazine*. September 15, 2013. http://nymag.com/thecut/2013/09/pill-no -prob-meet-the-pullout-generation.html

Grigg-Spall, Holly. *Sweetening the Pill: Or How We Got Hooked on Hormonal Birth Control*. Winchester, UK: Zero, 2013.

Jones, Rachel K., Julie Fennell, Jenny A. Higgins, and Kelly Blanchard. "Better than Nothing or Savvy Risk-Reduction Practice? The Importance of Withdrawal." *Contraception* 79.6 (2009): 407–10. https://www.guttmacher.org/sites /default/files/pdfs/pubs/journals/reprints/Contraception79-407-410.pdf

Killick, Stephen R., Christine Leary, James Trussell, and Katherine A. Guthrie. "Sperm Content of Pre-Ejaculatory Fluid." *Human Fertility* (Cambridge,

England) 14.1 (March 2011): 48–52. https://www.ncbi.nlm.nih.gov/pmc
/articles/PMC3564677/

Kuukasjarvi, Seppo, C.J. Peter Eriksson, Esa Koskela, Tapio Mappes, Kari
Nissinen, and Markus J. Rantala. "Attractiveness of Women's Body Odors
over the Menstrual Cycle: The Role of Oral Contraceptives and Receiver Sex."
Behavioral Ecology 15.4 (2004): 579–84. http://beheco.oxfordjournals.org
/content/15/4/579.short?rss=1&ssource=mfr

Northrup, Christiane. *Women's Bodies, Women's Wisdom: Creating Physical and
Emotional Health and Healing.* New York: Bantam, 2010.

Roach, Mary. *Bonk: The Curious Coupling of Science and Sex.* New York: W.W.
Norton, 2008.

Vitti, Alisa. *WomanCode: Perfect Your Cycle, Amplify Your Fertility, Supercharge
Your Sex Drive, and Become a Power Source.* San Francisco: HarperOne, 2013.

Wallwiener, Christian W., Lisa-Maria Wallwiener, Harald Seeger, Alfred O.
Mück, Johannes Bitzer, and Markus Wallwiener. "Prevalence of Sexual
Dysfunction and Impact of Contraception in Female German Medical
Students." *The Journal of Sexual Medicine* 7.6 (June 2010): 2139–148. https://
www.ncbi.nlm.nih.gov/pubmed/20487241

Weschler, Toni. *Taking Charge of Your Fertility: The Definitive Guide to Natural Birth
Control, Pregnancy Achievement, and Reproductive Health.* New York: Collins, 2006.

Zukerman, Zvi, David B. Weiss, and Raoul Orvieto. "Does Preejaculatory Penile
Secretion Originating from Cowper's Gland Contain Sperm?" *Journal of
Assisted Reproduction and Genetics* 20.4 (May 2003): 157–59 https://www.ncbi
.nlm.nih.gov/pubmed/12762415

EATER'S DIGEST: GUT CRITTERS AND THE SCOOP ON MY POOP

Blaser, Martin J. *Missing Microbes: How the Overuse of Antibiotics Is Fueling Our
Modern Plagues.* New York: Henry Holt and Co., 2014.

Biss, Eula. *On Immunity: An Inoculation.* Minneapolis, MN: Graywolf Press, 2014.

Chutkan, Robynne. *The Microbiome Solution: A Radical New Way to Heal Your Body
from the Inside Out.* New York: Avery, 2015.

Fujimura, Kei E., Tine Demoor, Marcus Rauch, Ali A. Faruqi, Sihyug Jang,
Christine C. Johnson, Homer A. Boushey, Edward Zoratti, Dennis Ownby,
Nicholas W. Lukacs, and Susan V. Lynch. "House Dust Exposure Mediates
Gut Microbiome *Lactobacillus* Enrichment and Airway Immune Defense against

Allergens and Virus Infection." *Proceedings of the National Academy of Sciences* 111.2 (June 2013): 805–10. http://www.pnas.org/content/111/2/805.abstract

Song, Se Jin, Christian Lauber, Elizabeth K. Costello, Catherine A. Lozupone, Gregory Humphrey, Donna Berg-Lyons, J. Gregory Caporaso, Dan Knights, Jose C. Clemente, Sara Nakielny, Jeffrey I. Gordon, Noah Fierer, and Rob Knight. "Cohabiting Family Members Share Microbiota with One Another and with Their Dogs." *eLife*. April 16, 2013. https://www.ncbi.nlm.nih.gov /pubmed/23599893

Sonnenburg, Justin, and Erica Sonnenburg. *The Good Gut: Taking Control of Your Weight, Your Mood, and Your Long-Term Health*. New York: Penguin Press, 2015.

RELAXATION STATION: LEARNING TO TAKE MY SOUL VITAMINS

Biziou, Barbara. *The Joy of Ritual: Spiritual Recipes to Celebrate Milestones, Ease Transitions, and Make Every Day Sacred*. New York: Golden, 1999.

Blackman, Andrew. "Can Money Buy You Happiness?" *The Wall Street Journal*. November 10, 2014. http://www.wsj.com/articles/can-money-buy-happiness -heres-what-science-has-to-say-1415569538

Cameron, Julia. *The Artist's Way: A Spiritual Path to Higher Creativity*. Los Angeles: Jeremy P. Tarcher/Perigee, 1992.

Elrod, Hal. *The Miracle Morning: The Not-So-Obvious Secret Guaranteed to Transform Your Life Before 8AM*. Hal Elrod International, 2014.

Orme-Johnson, S. W., and R. E. Herron, "Reduced Medical Care Utilization and Expenditures Through an Innovative Approach," Abstracts of the Association for Health Services Research 14th Annual Meeting, June 15–17, 1997, p. 19. https://www.ncbi.nlm.nih.gov/pubmed/10169245

Rodin, Judith, and E. J. Langer. "Long-Term Effects of a Control-Relevant Intervention with the Institutionalized Aged." *Journal of Personality and Social Psychology* 35.12 (December 1977): 897–902. https://www.ncbi.nlm.nih.gov /pubmed/592095

Williams, Mark, and Danny Penman. *Mindfulness: An Eight-Week Plan for Finding Peace in a Frantic World*. Emmaus, PA: Rodale, 2011.

EPILOGUE: CONNECTING THE DOTS

O'Rourke, Meghan. "What's Wrong with Me?" *The New Yorker*. November 20, 2015. http://www.newyorker.com/magazine/2013/08/26/whats-wrong-with-me